Overcoming Common Problems

Coping with Hearing Loss

CHRISTINE CRAGGS-HINTON

Library Learning Information

**Idea Store®
Whitechapel
321 Whitechapel Road
London E1 1BU**

020 7364 4332
www.ideastore.co.uk

Created and managed by
Tower Hamlets Council

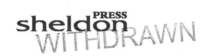

sheldon **PRESS**

WITHDRAWN

I would like to dedicate this book to my good friend Joann Holbrough, who has coped with hearing loss since childhood. I have never once heard Joann complain about her problem, and never once seen her retreat into the background because she couldn't catch all of a group conversation. I never realized until now just how much she has to contend with. She has my deepest admiration.

First published in Great Britain in 2007

Sheldon Press
36 Causton Street
London SW1P 4ST

British Library Cataloguing-in-Publication Data
A catalogue record for this book is available from the British Library

ISBN 978-1-84709-002-7

1 3 5 7 9 10 8 6 4 2

Typeset by Fakenham Photosetting Ltd, Fakenham, Norfolk
Printed and bound in Great Britain by Ashford Colour Press

Contents

About the author

CHRISTINE CRAGGS-HINTON, mother of three, followed a career in the Civil Service until, in 1991, she developed fibromyalgia, a chronic pain condition. Christine took up writing for therapeutic reasons and has, in the past few years, produced *Living with Fibromyalgia*, *The Fibromyalgia Healing Diet*, *The Chronic Fatigue Healing Diet*, *Coping with Polycystic Ovary Syndrome*, *Coping with Gout*, *How to Beat Pain*, *Coping with Eating Disorders and Body Image* and *Living with Multiple Sclerosis* (all published by Sheldon Press). She also writes for the Fibromyalgia Association UK and the related *FaMily* magazine. In recent years she has become interested in fiction writing, too.

Introduction

I had no idea just how much being hard of hearing impinged on a person's life until I began researching this book. Indeed, I imagine that most people with normal hearing have no concept at all of the emotional turmoil experienced by so many affected individuals. Some hearing people would surely not treat the hearing impaired with such insensitivity and irritation if they understood just a fraction of what those with loss of hearing go through. Yet this is incredibly common, particularly in the over-60s age group. It's also becoming more prevalent, affecting people at increasingly younger ages. Recently, I was shocked to read that 60 per cent of freshmen entering a US university were found to have hearing loss, and that of that number, 14 per cent had hearing similar to that of the average 65-year-old.

Communication is a large part of what the human being is all about, but it's made incredibly difficult by not always hearing what is said to you or, in fact, regularly mishearing it. The inability to communicate effectively often leads to stress, low mood, reduced confidence, decreased self-esteem and feelings of isolation. It doesn't help that hearing loss can also be accompanied by problems such as headaches, dizziness, nausea and tinnitus (ringing or roaring sounds in the head).

As well as hearing at a reduced volume, many people with impaired hearing perceive speech sounds that are distorted or unclear, making them even more difficult to understand. Individuals with mild to moderate hearing loss may not even be fully aware of their problem – particularly if its onset was very gradual. When they constantly misunderstand what is said they may even think they are growing 'senile' or have a terrible mental condition for which there's no cure. It may be family and friends who eventually point out what's really happening.

With more severe hearing loss, individuals usually know they are being spoken to, but what they actually hear is an indecipherable mumble. They may be able to use speechreading to guess at what was said – largely by lipreading, facial expressions, gestures and the odd heard word. Even so, they are likely to misunderstand frequently, their response causing either disdain, mystified frowns or absolute hilarity. Few of the hearing impaired have not been looked on as fools or simpletons at some time in their lives, which is something many continually dread. It can even make the person retreat into a shell and not even bother trying to communicate.

This book discusses the chief causes of hearing problems and aims to help you cope with their practical implications in different situations. It also offers a number of strategies that should help you to communicate more effectively. Hearing aids, cochlea implants, sound amplification devices and so on are discussed, as is hearing therapy and the complementary therapies reported to be useful for treating hearing loss and tinnitus.

You may feel alone and isolated with your problem, but please feel assured that hearing loss is widespread. A lot can be done to alleviate it, on both a practical and psychological level. You can make a start by reading this book.

1

Why can't I hear properly?

Hearing loss has been calculated to be the most common disability in the Western world – and the number of cases is rising all the time. Indeed, it's said that few people are not touched in some way by the inability to hear normally, whether it's a problem for a close family member or friend, or whether they suffer from it themselves.

Hearing loss – also referred to as deafness, being hard of hearing or hearing impairment – is defined as the decreased ability to discriminate sounds, and may be either a temporary or a permanent condition. It is one of the most common disorders to affect middle-aged and elderly people, and can be hereditary, or caused by disease, infection, medications, trauma or prolonged exposure to loud noise.

According to the Royal National Institute for Deaf People (RNID), there are an estimated nine million deaf and partially hearing people in the UK, of whom 673,000 are profoundly deaf. The majority of these individuals will have lost their hearing gradually with increasing age. Surprisingly, age-related hearing loss can first occur in a person aged 40, which is not that old nowadays. Of people aged 60 and over, approximately a third suffer from hearing problems, and of people aged 80 and over, more than half are affected.

Each person with hearing loss will hear a quality of sound that differs from that of another person with hearing loss. For instance, one individual may only be able to hear very high-pitched noises, such as a fire or smoke alarm, a new baby's cries, soprano singing, certain power tools and the squeals and shrieks of children. Another may also be able to hear a ringing telephone and the voices of women and children. Yet another may be able to hear only low-pitched sounds such as drum beats, male voices and the bass notes in music. The volume of hearing can also vary immensely, ranging from difficulty following speech – especially against background noise – to being unable to hear anything at all without the aid of a hearing device or sound amplification system.

No other prevalent condition socially alienates a person more than hearing loss. Many people believe blindness to be the most isolating disorder, and admittedly blind people are unable to appreciate colour, texture and tone; they may not even be able to see their family and friends. Yet they can still communicate, still be a part of a social group. Moreover, they can still be themselves – particularly with people they know well. Individuals with hearing loss, on the other hand, feel socially excluded and may change from being relaxed and outgoing to being introverted, irritable and depressed – even with their nearest and dearest.

Because people with hearing loss can have trouble understanding their GP's advice, hearing someone creep up behind them, responding to warnings, hearing doorbells and alarms (including fire and smoke alarms), life can be very difficult, even dangerous. Hearing loss also makes it problematic for individuals concerned to enjoy chatting with family and friends. The ability to communicate is an essential requirement of human society. We are social beings who gain feelings of acceptance and self-worth from our interactions with others. When hearing loss makes it difficult to communicate effectively, we can feel isolated and our self-esteem can plummet.

To some extent, hearing loss is another disease of Western civilization. When recently a Sudanese tribe living deep in the African bush were studied, it was discovered that at any age they had better hearing than a comparable group of farmers in the West. More significantly, the older members of the tribe could hear as well as the younger members. It was always believed that hearing loss 'just happens' with age and that it was partly due to the loss of certain cells in the inner ear, together with reduced blood circulation in the head. However, studies such as the one mentioned above indicate that noxious influences throughout life can also affect hearing. Such influences include noise trauma and the toxicity of certain drugs and medications – both of which are discussed in this book.

Sound and the ear

When a person is hard of hearing, something about the ear and auditory system is not working as well as it should. The functioning ear is a remarkable organ, but a great deal can go wrong. When it's working properly, it picks up all the sounds close by and translates the information into a form that the brain can readily comprehend.

To understand the way the ear functions, it is important first to know what sound is.

The basics of hearing

Sound travels through the air as vibrations in the form of waves. To hear sound, the ear has to direct the sound waves to the hearing part of the ear and convert them into an electrical signal the brain can understand. Once these signals reach the brain, the signals are translated into meaningful information, such as language or music, with qualities such as pitch and volume.

The outer ear

The ear (see Figure 1) is divided into three parts: the outer ear, the middle ear and the inner ear. The skin and cartilage that are visible on the outside of the head make up the outer ear and are known as the *pinna* and ear canal – the latter of which extends about 2.5 cm (one inch) into the head. The pinna acts as a collector of sound. It is not so efficient in the human as in some animals, however. For instance, a dog's mobile ears point in the direction of the sound and a fox has such a large pinna that, when it listens intently, it can even hear ants moving underground.

The ear canal has two prime functions.

- It protects the fragile eardrum from the elements.
- Using *resonance*, it amplifies the pitches that are important for understanding speech. (It is resonance that amplifies the sound of your breath when you blow over the top of a bottle.)

The middle ear

Sound waves travel along the ear canal where they vibrate the *tympanic membrane*, commonly called the eardrum – a highly sensitive structure. This is a thin, cone-shaped piece of tissue that is positioned between the ear canal and the middle ear. The middle ear is connected to the throat via the Eustachian tube. Air from the atmosphere flows in through the ear as well as through the mouth, and air pressure on both sides of the eardrum should be equal. This balance of pressure allows the eardrum to vibrate when hit by a sound wave. The vibration is rapidly conveyed to the middle ear, which consists of three bones called *ossicles*, the smallest bones in the body. They include the hammer (*malleus*), the anvil (*incus*) and the stirrup (*stapes*). The ossicles compress the movements in the eardrum, so that all the vibration is focused on the tiny footplate of the stirrup, which transmits the movements to the inner ear.

The inner ear

The inner ear is effectively made up of two organs called the *cochlea* (the Latin word for snail) and the *semicircular canals* (or *labyrinth*), and the endings of the auditory nerve. The cochlea is the most complex part of the ear, for its job is to convert the vibrations that are passed

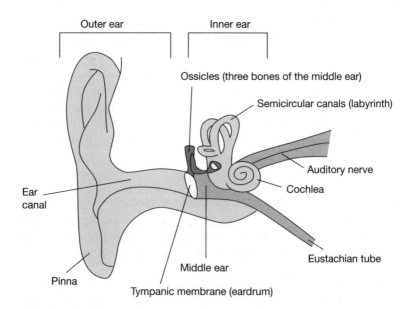

Figure 1 The ear

from the ossicles into electrical information the brain can recognize as sound. The cochlea achieves this by means of the many tiny hair cells that move in response to the vibrations, generating an electrical signal that is relayed to the brain via the auditory nerve. (The semicircular canals are concerned with balance rather than hearing.)

Hearing loss measured

A person's sensitivity to sound is measured in decibels. As the mathematical definition of a decibel is complicated, here are some approximate decibel measurements to help demonstrate its meaning:

- 10 decibels – normal breathing
- 20 decibels – a whisper or leaves rustling in a breeze
- 45 decibels – ordinary conversational speech
- 55 decibels – loud conversational speech
- 85 decibels – a vacuum cleaner, city traffic or a tube station
- 95 decibels – a lawnmower
- 105 decibels – a video arcade or factory with loud machinery
- 110 decibels – a symphony concert or motorcycle – hearing may become painful at this level
- 113 decibels – a personal music player headset
- 115 decibels – a chain saw or in the audience of a loud amplified rock band
- 127 decibels – a football game, in the stadium – above 120 decibels is considered temporarily deafening
- 135 decibels – a pneumatic drill – above 135 decibels, hearing will become extremely painful and hearing loss may result if exposure is prolonged
- 157 decibels – a balloon bursting
- 162 decibels – fireworks, at a range of three feet
- 170 decibels – a shotgun being fired
- 180 decibels – an aircraft taking off at close range – above 180 decibels, eventual hearing loss is almost certain with even short-term exposure

As a loss of hearing can also be measured in decibels, it's possible to see how particular decibel loss is likely to affect communication. For instance, a person with a 45 decibel loss will struggle to hear and comprehend ordinary conversational speech – it will translate as the softest sound a healthy ear can detect. On the other hand, a person with a 55 decibel loss will barely be able to hear and comprehend loud conversational speech. It can be seen, then, that over 45 decibels, a small decibel loss can make a huge difference. That's why, if you already suffer from hearing loss, it's important to avoid damaging your hearing further, through exposure to loud noises in particular.

A hearing loss of 1–15 decibels is not considered a problem. However, the following decibel losses create the problems described below:

- 16–25 – minimal hearing loss. Problems will arise in noisy surroundings, such as at a party with loud music. Faint or distant speech may cause a problem.
- 26–40 – mild hearing loss. With no background noise, the person may be able to communicate very well. In the presence of background noise, or if the speaker is some distance away, speech will be difficult to hear. Moreover, the person is likely to miss up to 50 per cent of a group discussion. Use of a hearing aid in certain situations can make a lot of difference (see Chapter 4 for coping strategies, Chapter 5 for a hearing therapy programme and Chapter 6 for information and advice on hearing aids).
- 41–55 – moderate hearing loss. Conversation without background noise can be heard up to five feet away, but may not be completely understood. At more than five feet away, very little of the conversation will be understood.
- 56–70 – moderate to severe hearing loss. Without the use of sound amplification, only very loud speech will be heard and understood. Very little can be heard and understood in group situations. The ability to speechread will be useful (see Chapter 5 for information and advice on speechreading).
- 71–90 – severe hearing loss. Only loud speech at very close quarters – such as one foot away – will be heard, as well as loud bangs and explosions. Moreover, loud speech is usually distorted, making comprehension difficult. People affected will not even be able to hear themselves speaking. Sound amplification by

means of a hearing aid or cochlea implant is necessary, as well as training in speechreading, speech therapy and so on.

- 91 and above – profound deafness. Occasional very loud sounds may be heard or felt through vibration. In the main, the person must depend on vision instead of hearing for the processing of information. A cochlea implant may be helpful. Training in speechreading, speech therapy and knowledge of sign language can make a great difference, however.

Whether your hearing is already damaged or not, sound intensities of over 90 decibels – or lower when exposure is prolonged and repeated – can cause permanent damage to the ear. Higher intensities can only be handled for short bursts of time before irreparable damage results. Extremely loud sounds – from sudden explosions, for example – can even cause the eardrum to rupture.

Conductive hearing loss (CHL)

Because the hearing system is incredibly complex, a variety of problems can arise. The type of hearing loss experienced is categorized by the location in which the problem lies within the auditory system. For instance, a person with damage within the outer ear canal has *conductive* hearing loss; a person with damage to the inner ear has *sensorineural* hearing loss, and a person with damage to the nerve that transmits messages from the cochlea to the brain has *neural* hearing loss. A fourth type, called 'mixed', is simply a combination of conductive and sensorineural hearing loss.

Conductive hearing loss is caused by poor transmission of sound waves through the outer ear canal to the eardrum and the tiny bones – called ossicles – of the middle ear. A person with conductive hearing loss will normally experience poor transmission of sound waves to the inner ear, and be less able to hear faint sounds. In many cases, conductive hearing loss can be corrected by medical or surgical means.

In the over-55 age group, conductive hearing loss occurs in 25 per cent of men and 19 per cent of women. Causative conditions may include the following:

Age-related deterioration

As people age, their hearing can gradually deteriorate – the scientific term for this problem is *presbyacusis*. The deterioration can be caused by several factors, which often work in unison. For a start, just as the knees and shoulders can stiffen with age, so can the tiny joints between the ossicles of the ear, as well as those within the cochlea. Hair cells in the cochlea are commonly affected by wear and tear too, becoming less mobile and even breaking off as the person gets older. The pathways of the nerves involved in hearing are also likely to degenerate over time, meaning the signal might not be effectively transmitted to the brain.

If you think or know you are suffering from age-related hearing loss, you may wonder why most of your friends of the same age still have good hearing. Some people are genetically disposed to having problems with their hearing, in the same way as some are disposed to developing arthritis and some to developing high blood pressure. In other words, the tendency to have the problem runs in the family. Prolonged exposure to noise or exposure to sudden loud sounds such as bangs and explosions can also precipitate hearing impairment. You can halt further damage by avoiding loud noises or by using good ear protection. In addition – and quite surprisingly – an individual's general health throughout their lives is now known to affect their hearing.

Because hearing loss most commonly occurs with advancing years, its incidence is increasing as the population becomes proportionately older. Unfortunately, hearing loss is strongly connected with the ageing process, so can still carry a stigma. Many people fear getting older, and some cope with the fear by looking with disdain at the signs of ageing. No one wants their eyesight to deteriorate, their joints to stiffen, their teeth to rot – neither do they want their hearing to decline. Young people wear glasses as well as older people, sight problems are not so linked with ageing. Stiff joints are not generally so obvious; our modern dentists can counter tooth decay – but there's no such help for age-related hearing loss. Indeed, being over 50 and using a hearing aid seems only to proclaim to the world that you are wearing out. Hearing aids can be a terrific bonus if you know how to use one properly, but the stigma remains.

Although age-related damage to hearing is permanent, medical and surgical interventions can help in some people. As this book is largely concerned with age-related hearing loss, we will return to the subject many more times.

Infection in the ear canal

When conductive hearing loss is caused by *otitis*, a bacterial infection of the middle ear, inflammation and perforation of the eardrum can occur. Perforation, where a hole appears in the eardrum, generally allows mucus fluid to drain out of the ear canal and allows bacteria to enter, causing further infection. A perforated eardrum can also be caused by injury.

Infection in the middle ear

Most childhood earaches and infections – called *otitis media* – arise in the space behind the eardrum (the middle ear). These painful infections can also occur in adults. Otitis media means that inflammation in the throat from a cold virus can cause the 'plugged' sensation you get in your ears. The inflammation restricts the opening of the Eustachian tube, preventing air from travelling up it and causing a slight vacuum in the middle ear. The vacuum draws fluid from the tissues into the middle ear, causing some hearing loss. If the fluid becomes infected, otitis media is the result.

Glue ear

Four out of every five pre-school children suffer from glue ear – a collection of fluid in the middle ear resulting from colds, ear infections and allergies. Glue ear can cause not only some temporary hearing loss, but can also lead to dizziness and vomiting. It can be treated by use of medications or, in severe cases, by the surgical application of grommets.

Very few adults experience glue ear, but it can occur. An adult with glue ear lasting more than a few days will normally need specialist advice and should see their GP.

Impacted earwax

The purpose of natural wax – *cerumen* – in the ear canal is to trap dust and other particles so they don't damage the middle and inner ear. We are told that, ideally, we should not have to clean our ear canals – that they are, in fact, self-cleaning, the wax falling out of the ear in minuscule grains with the trapped particles. Unfortunately, some people have too little earwax, which causes dry, itchy ears and even infection. In others too much wax accumulates, preventing sound from travelling through the ear canal as well as it should.

Over-the-counter products such as Debrox and Murine ear drops may soften the wax. If not, you should visit your doctor. It's important that you know whether or not you have a perforation in your eardrum, as if you have, earwax softeners can cause an infection. Some people are very sensitive to earwax softeners and may develop a rash, pain or tenderness. If this happens to you, you should stop using softeners immediately.

If you think you have too much earwax, you should see your doctor. He or she will be able to wash out, vacuum or remove any excess wax with special instruments. You should never use such things as cotton buds, hairclips (bobby pins) or twisted serviette corners to clean out your ears. Pushing anything into your ear canal serves only to push the wax in deeper and impact it further. Moreover, the skin of the ear canal is very easily injured, and the eardrum is just as easily perforated.

The presence of a foreign body

A foreign body lodged in the ear canal will obviously prevent some sound waves from travelling to the eardrum and ossicles, restricting hearing. Children are renowned for pushing tiny items into their ears, sometimes causing damage in the process. When this happens, they should be taken to the A & E department of their local hospital for the item to be removed. In most cases, this can be easily achieved by the use of surgical instruments.

Otosclerosis

Otosclerosis is characterized by the abnormal growth of bone within the middle ear that stops the ossicles from vibrating and so prevents some sound from reaching the inner ear. With this condition, hearing loss is progressive, but profound deafness does not result.

Otosclerosis can cause different types of hearing loss, depending on which structure in the middle ear is affected – it generally arises in the stapes. The condition can also cause tinnitus (sensations of ringing or tapping in the ears), dizziness, nausea and balance problems. One ear may be targeted first of all, but the condition usually spreads to the second ear.

Research has shown that risk factors for otosclerosis include the following:

- women are more likely to have it than men;
- it generally arises between the ages of 15 and 30;
- Caucasian (white) people are most commonly affected;
- it tends to run in families, so there is clearly a genetic factor;
- if one parent has otosclerosis, the child has a 25 per cent chance of developing the disorder. If both parents have it, the risk goes up to 50 per cent;
- susceptible women can develop the condition during pregnancy, due to hormonal changes;
- it can result from a viral infection, such as measles and mumps;
- evidence suggests that drinking non-fluoridated water may increase the risk of developing otosclerosis in susceptible people.

In some people, the use of a hearing aid can boost hearing sufficiently. If not, surgical treatment includes the removal of the affected area and replacement with a prosthesis or artificial stapes.

Rheumatoid arthritis

Rheumatoid arthritis is a chronic inflammatory disease affecting the joints and surrounding muscles, tendons, ligaments and blood vessels. In rare cases, the inflammation can attack the joints between the ossicles, causing pain and varying degrees of hearing loss. Drug therapy with salicylates, which decrease inflammation and relieve joint pain, can improve the problem, as can the use of non-steroidal anti-inflammatory drugs such as ibuprofen, naproxen and diclofenac.

Other abnormalities

Problems such as faulty Eustachian tube function can cause hearing impairment, as can malformation or absence of the outer ear, ear canal or middle ear. Benign tumours in the middle ear are a rare condition, but do develop in some people. However, they are accompanied by other medical conditions as well as hearing loss.

Sensorineural hearing loss (SNHL)

This type of hearing loss arises when the tiny hair cells in the inner ear (cochlea) are damaged or destroyed, or when there is damage to the nerve pathways that run from the inner ear to the brain. SNHL is sometimes called 'nerve deafness', a term that is not entirely accurate as it wrongly excludes damage to the hair cells.

Twenty-three per cent of the population over 65 are affected by SNHL. Unfortunately, this type of hearing loss is permanent, so cannot be corrected by medical or surgical means. However, it doesn't always signal profound deafness. The individual may be able to hear muffled sounds.

Some people have reported that the use of particular complementary therapies has improved their SNHL (see Chapter 8).

Loudness recruitment

A widespread problem with SNHL is known as 'loudness recruitment' (also called reduced dynamic range of hearing). This means that loud sounds may be heard in just the same way as they are heard by someone with normal hearing, but you may not be able to hear soft sounds unless they are made louder. If both loud and soft sounds were made louder, simply by turning up the volume on your TV or stereo, for example, you would find the loud sounds uncomfortable to listen to. This type of problem does not affect people with conductive hearing loss.

If you would like someone close with normal hearing to know what loudness recruitment is like, you could ask them to listen to orchestral music on a personal stereo in a noisy place, such as on an underground train, close to roadworks and so on. When they turn up the volume to hear the quiet sections of music, the sudden loud sections will be uncomfortable to listen to. Of course, people with normal hearing have the option of turning down the volume immediately, which people with SNHL have not. In quiet surroundings, people with normal hearing can turn down the volume and still hear the wide range of sounds comfortably, which again people with SNHL cannot.

As well as age-related wear and tear (as discussed above), the possible causes of SNHL include:

Noise-induced deafness (acoustic trauma)

If there's one main feature of youth culture in the West, it's loud music – very loud music. It will be hardly surprising, then, to learn that the fastest-growing group suffering from noise-induced hearing loss is teenagers, due to the extra-loud music they play.

Pete Townsend of The Who was one of the champions of ear-splitting music, ending his shows with a screaming explosion of feedback and amplified racket as he smashed his guitar to pieces at full volume. Nowadays, he is hard of hearing and a supporter of the charity HEAR (Hearing Education and Awareness for Rockers). HEAR was founded by Kathy Peck, who played amplified rock in the USA for several years until, in her early 20s, she developed severe hearing loss. Sixty per cent of our early rock and roll giants are now hard of hearing.

Loud music isn't the only threat to hearing, however. In our modern industrialized world our ears are assaulted from all sides by urban traffic, motorways, aeroplanes, lawnmowers, office and factory machinery, PA systems and so on. Prolonged exposure to such noise eventually takes its toll, as does exposure to loud bangs and explosions – all these things cause trauma to the hair cells within the ear. The cells are effectively battered around by violent sound waves, many even being broken off by the force of the resulting terrific vibrations. Individuals who already have hearing impairment are likely to be highly susceptible to acoustic trauma and should be very wary of exposure to noise.

If you can answer 'yes' to any of the following, you are being overexposed to noise:

- Do you regularly need to raise your voice to talk above a noise?

- Do you have a ringing or roaring sensation after the exposure to noise?
- Do you have difficulty hearing normal conversations for a while after the exposure?

When the Medical Research Council (MRC), in a 1997–8 survey, compared the symptoms of people working in a noisy environment with those working in a non-noisy environment, it was estimated that over half a million were suffering from noise-induced hearing loss. However, in 2001, the Department for Work and Pensions (DWP) used a ten per cent sample of their records to estimate that only 14,000 people were in receipt of disablement pension for occupational deafness. Many of the individuals in the MRC survey will not have met the DWP criterion of at least 50 decibels of hearing loss to be eligible for benefit. This equates to a 20 per cent disability – a substantial impairment. The present criteria also call for an employee to have worked in specified noisy conditions for a minimum of ten years. Since 1997 there has been a distinct downward trend of new cases receiving disablement benefit for occupational deafness, which we can only hope is due to employers being more careful to follow guidelines for noise levels in the workplace. There are also fewer mills and factories.

According to DWP records, the people who were newly awarded benefit in 2004 worked in the following industries:

- energy extraction and water supply (9.9 cases per 100,000 employees)
- manufacturing (5.1 cases per 100,000 employees)
- construction (3.8 cases per 100,000 employees)

If you are exposed to loud noise in the workplace, it's important that you wear hearing protection such as muffs or proper earplugs. With essential exposure, take regular breaks from the noise to allow the hair cells in your ears to recover. People with hearing impairment who work in a noisy environment would be best advised to find a job in quieter conditions. Changing your job is a big deal, but not so big as experiencing a far greater deterioration in your hearing.

Experts predict that the recent leap in sales of portable music players such as personal stereos, MP3 players and iPods will give rise to many more cases of noise-induced hearing loss in the future. Indeed, the Royal National Institute for Deaf People has urged individuals to avoid listening to music through their headphones with the volume turned up high. In a survey, they found that 39 per cent of 18- to 24-year-olds listened to music through headphones for at least an hour every day, and 42 per cent admitted they thought the volume was too high. According to the RNID, hearing is threatened at 80 decibels, yet some MP3 players can reach 105 decibels. iPods manufactured in the European Union have a built-in sound limiter to comply with noise safety levels, but some individuals are removing that.

If you listen to a portable music player on high volume for regular prolonged periods, you would be best advised either to turn down the volume or have frequent breaks in between listening. If you hear ringing or buzzing in your ears after using the player, it's a sure sign that the volume was too high. Many high street stores now sell protective filters for in-ear headphones.

If you frequent nightclubs, it's advisable to give your ears a rest by taking regular breaks from the noisy dance floor – chill-out areas are usually available. DJs, musicians and regular clubbers can lower their risk by wearing soft foam or plastic ear plugs – it isn't enough to stuff bits of tissue or cotton wool into your ears. Indeed, Kathy Peck, who set up the HEAR charity, recommends that people always wear earplugs when attending rock concerts. It's also advisable to keep as far away as possible from the loudspeakers.

Ménière's disease

Ménière's disease (also called *endolymphatic hydrops*) is a common problem where the fluid volume in the semicircular canals of the inner ear is too great, leading to elevated pressure levels. This causes attacks of nausea and dizziness, the latter of which feels like violent spinning and whirling. During an attack, dizzy spells may last for several hours at a time, and the individual's sense of balance will be so impaired that he or she is highly likely to accidentally bump into furniture, door jambs and so on, becoming covered in bruises. Fortunately, there are certain sedative drugs that can combat the dizziness.

In the early stages of the disorder, hearing in the low ranges will usually deteriorate during an attack, but should return to normal or near normal when the attack is over. The frequency of episodes varies from person to person, but will usually recur several times over the duration of the illness. Hearing loss may even fail to recover fully after an episode. If the disease continues over several years, hearing loss is generally constant and irreversible. Anxiety, depression and loss of confidence often result. However, as stated earlier, whatever the cause of your hearing loss, you can find help in this book, as well as from audiologists and hearing therapists.

Infection or inflammation of the brain or its covering

The viral infections meningitis and encephalitis can damage the inner ear and result in hearing loss. The former causes inflammation of the covering of the brain – the meninges – whereas the latter causes inflammation of the brain itself.

Certain medications

In rare cases, very high doses of certain medications can temporarily have an adverse effect on the hair cells. These medications include aspirin, quinine and some powerful antibiotics. Medication-induced hearing loss is usually preceded by tinnitus. If such symptoms develop, you should consult your doctor, who may be able to change your prescription.

This type of hearing loss will normally improve once you stop taking the medication responsible. However, it isn't always possible to change the drug – where there is a life-threatening infection or when using particular chemotherapy drugs. In such instances, you really have no choice but to take the medication and accept the hearing shortfall.

Multiple sclerosis (MS)

About six per cent of individuals with MS suffer from hearing impairment, making it a fairly rare symptom. The deficit in hearing generally takes place during an acute exacerbation of MS (known as a relapse), when separated from a previous exacerbation by at least one month. In MS, the problem arises when the nerves involved in hearing become inflamed.

Viral infections of the auditory nerve

When hearing loss is sudden, the most common reason is a viral infection, which can cause inflammation of the inner ear or auditory nerve. Apart from the sudden deficit in hearing, the person experiences no pain, fever, muscle cramps or other signs of a viral illness. Occasionally, signs of an upper respiratory infection may precede the onset of sudden SNHL. *Cytomegalovirus* (CMV) is a common congenital viral infection associated with a number of neurological disorders, including hearing loss.

A metabolic imbalance

In rare cases, abnormal hormone levels in disorders such as diabetes and thyroid problems can cause some hearing loss. When hormone levels are normalized with the use of medications, hearing is normally restored.

A brain tumour

Benign and malignant tumours can damage the nerves involved in hearing, leading to some hearing loss.

Sensitivity and discrimination

SNHL generally involves a combination of sensitivity and discrimination problems. For example, reduced sensitivity causes the person to have difficulty detecting soft sounds, such as someone whispering, a bird singing and the rush of water in a stream. When the whispering becomes louder, the bird and brook closer, the sound may be detected and correctly interpreted. Discrimination problems refer to a difficulty distinguishing one sound from another and the inability to understand speech. Some people suffer from both sensitivity and discrimination problems and find that even when speech is loud enough for them to hear, the sounds are so distorted they can't immediately recognize it as speech.

Sensitivity

An individual with sensitivity problems will have more difficulty hearing the higher frequencies than the lower frequencies (pitches) – even when hearing loss is mild. For example, the high-pitched consonants f, s, t, v, ch, sh, th, k, z, and p are formed by air hissing or bursting from the mouth. An ear that can't properly pick up these sounds will have trouble with comprehension, meaning that words like thigh, sigh, shy, tie and pie may sound exactly the same. The person must look at the context of the sentence before deducing what the word was. Of course, when consonants are not heard clearly all the time, the chore of working them out from the context becomes tiring and before long the gist of the entire speech is lost. This is where speechreading comes in very handy (see Chapter 5, which deals with speechreading).

Discrimination

As stated above, discrimination refers to the ability to tell one sound apart from another. Discrimination problems are measured by ascertaining the percentage of a list of one-syllable words that are correctly recognized when introduced at a normal level of sound. It's far more difficult to discern individual words than ones presented in conversation because there's no frame of reference. The score a patient is given relates to the number of words they repeat correctly and reflects their ability to understand speech under optimal listening conditions. A normal score ranges from 90 to 100 per cent.

The following describes the ability to discriminate words at specific percentages of discrimination loss:

- 75–90 per cent. There are not so many undeciphered words that this person cannot guess the correct words in most situations.
- 60–75 per cent. For this person, speech is frequently distorted and he or she has difficulty following a conversation.
- 45–60 per cent. For this person, communication is difficult without speechreading to fill in the gaps.
- Below 45 per cent. This person is unable to decipher normal speech and must rely on other techniques to communicate effectively.

2

Identifying hearing loss

Not everyone is conscious of his or her hearing impairment, particularly if it has crept up very slowly – most people with hearing loss experience gradual deterioration. Some individuals simply don't realize they're having to turn up the volume on their TVs, radios and stereo systems, and it doesn't register why they often misunderstand speech. This doesn't mean they're not very switched on – not at all. When something happens so gradually, perhaps over several years, it's easy to dismiss it as a problem or not even think about it at all.

Questions to ask yourself

For an indication of whether you have a hearing problem, ask yourself the following questions:

- Is it a strain to follow a conversation?
- Is it particularly difficult to follow a conversation when two or more people are talking?
- Do I tune out when more than one person is talking?
- After a long conversation, do I often feel tired and irritable?
- Do most of the people I speak to seem to mumble, or not speak very clearly?
- Do I regularly ask people to repeat what they have said?
- Does it seem that my friends and family avoid conversations with me?
- Do some people seem baffled or even embarrassed by my answers to their questions?
- Is it difficult to hear when there is noise in the background?
- Do I have trouble hearing on the telephone?
- Do people complain that I turn up the TV volume too high?
- Do I sometimes not hear the doorbell or telephone ringing?

- Am I sometimes confused about where sounds are coming from?
- Do I find it particularly hard to hear women and children?
- Am I troubled with ringing, roaring or hissing in my ears?
- Are some sounds uncomfortably loud?

If you can answer 'yes' to one or more of the above questions, you are likely to have some degree of hearing loss.

There is one last question that is of even more significance. Ask a family member to answer this:

- Do you think this person is suffering from hearing loss?

What should I do?

Because hearing loss is a serious problem, the best thing you can do, if you appear to have a problem, is visit your GP. He or she may be able to identify the problem and prescribe the appropriate treatment. If not, you can expect to be referred to an *otolaryngologist* – a doctor (and surgeon) who specializes in disorders of the ear, nose, throat, head and neck.

The otolaryngologist will ask lots of questions about your difficulties with hearing, including whether other family members have any hearing impairment. You will also undergo a thorough examination and your hearing may be tested. If a clear picture of your problem is formed, the otolaryngologist should be able to give a diagnosis and offer a choice of treatment options. If not, you are likely to be referred to an audiologist – another professional in the field of hearing (see below).

Other problems linked to the auditory system

If you have a problem with balance (vertigo), ringing in your ears, earache or excessive wax, you should see your GP. If he or she isn't able to treat it, you may be referred to the appropriate professional.

Seeing an audiologist

An audiologist will most likely test your hearing to determine where the problem is located. First, however, he or she will ask you a few questions about past illnesses, any medications you are taking, loud noises you have been exposed to and whether you have ever incurred physical damage to your ear(s).

The audiologist's next step is likely to be to look into your ear with a cone-shaped instrument with a light in one end – this is called an otoscope. It helps the audiologist to see whether there are any abnormalities in the ear canal or eardrum.

The pure-tone tests

For the pure-tone tests, you will be taken to a quiet room and either given headphones to place over your ears or a pair of soft foam ear plugs to use. The headphones or plugs will deliver into your ears a series of 'pure tones' that vary in frequency and volume. You will show that you have heard a tone by either pressing a button or raising your hand. The audiologist will plot the softest sounds you can hear on an audiogram.

Following this, the audiologist will place a small bone conductor behind each ear and run through the pure-tone test again. The bone conductor transmits sound to the cochlea (in the inner ear), effectively bypassing the middle and outer ear. This test helps the audiologist to determine the type of hearing loss you have.

Speech tests

Speech tests are the next step. Once again you will be seated in a quiet room, with the audiologist in an adjacent room. He or she will then ask you to repeat words of two syllables that become increasingly softer. You will then be asked to repeat words of one syllable, delivered at the same volume. This is called the speech discrimination, or word recognition, score. It allows the audiologist to calculate the volume at which you can detect and understand speech.

Middle ear tests

The audiologist may also decide to check your middle ear, inserting a probe into your ear and increasing then decreasing the air pressure while a tone is played to you through the headphones or plugs. Several frequencies may be played to you, allowing the acoustic reflex to be measured for each and providing excellent information regarding the function of your middle ear.

The audiologist may also place a soft plug into your ear canal to measure the movement of the eardrum and middle ear system. This procedure helps to detect dysfunction in the eardrum, middle ear bones or Eustachian tube.

Test results

The results of the above hearing tests are recorded on a chart called an audiogram. It will show the frequencies at which your hearing is worst, which ear you hear better in, and how severe your hearing loss is.

The audiologist should then take the time to explain your test results fully. If you don't understand something, or have further questions, it's important that you ask. You have a right to know. Unanswered questions can cause a build-up of stress. If you think of something after your visit, ask your doctor if you can make another appointment to see the audiologist, as early as possible.

See Chapter 5 for information on hearing therapy from an audiologist or other hearing specialist.

Specialized audiometric testing

If your case history and test results warrant further testing, there are specialized tests the audiologist may like to perform. They are as follows:

Auditory brainstem response (diagnostic ABR)

If there is a significant difference between the hearing in your left and right ears, the diagnostic ABR test may be used. This test can assess the auditory system at the level of the brainstem. To carry out the test, you will have electrodes attached to your forehead, each earlobe and the top of your head. Earphones will also be placed in your ear canals. You will be asked to lie on a bed and try to relax – some people fall asleep during the test, which is fine, for it helps the audiologist to analyse the information gathered and to compare the results from each ear.

Threshold ABR

Some people are not able to provide accurate hearing responses for the pure-tone testing procedure, in which case threshold ABR may take place. The approach is the same as for diagnostic ABR, except that the audiologist is now looking for the softest level that a response can be obtained. A range of stimuli can be used, such as clicks and frequency-specific tone-bursts.

Electrocochleography (ECoG)

This test is much like the diagnostic ABR test, except that an electrode is placed near the eardrum by an otologist. This test measures the electrical responses in the inner ear. It can be useful for detecting such disorders as Meniere's disease.

Otoacoustic emissions (OAEs)

Cochlea outer hair cell function can be detected by this test, and may be recommended when hearing loss occurs suddenly, when you are taking a certain medication, or when there is a difference in hearing between your ears. To perform this test, the audiologist will place a probe into your ear canal and assess your response to a series of tones.

The diagnosis

Three components must be taken into account before a clear picture of your hearing condition can be drawn. They are as follows:

- the type of hearing loss, as covered in Chapter 1;
- the degree of hearing loss, as discussed below;
- the configuration of the hearing loss, as discussed below.

The degree of hearing loss

The degree of hearing loss means the severity of the problem. The categories used to determine the degree are as follows:

- normal range or no impairment;
- mild loss;
- moderate loss;

- severe loss;
- profound loss.

The configuration of the hearing loss

The configuration of the problem refers to the extent of the deficit at each frequency and the overall picture of hearing created. A configuration showing poor hearing in the lower frequencies and good hearing in the higher frequencies would be described as low-frequency loss. On the other hand, poor hearing in the higher tones and good hearing in the lower tones would be referred to as high-frequency loss. Some individuals experience the same amount of hearing loss for low and high tones.

Other descriptions of hearing problems include the following:

- Bilateral versus unilateral. With bilateral hearing loss, both ears are affected, whereas with unilateral loss, only one ear is affected.
- Symmetrical versus asymmetrical. Symmetrical hearing means that the degree of loss and configuration are the same in each ear.
- Progressive versus sudden hearing loss. Progressive hearing loss is the gradual deterioration of hearing over time. Sudden hearing loss occurs quickly and requires immediate medical attention.
- Fluctuating versus stable hearing loss. In some cases, hearing loss fluctuates, sometimes improving, sometimes worsening, such as in Ménière's disease. In most cases, however, hearing loss is stable.

3

Adjusting to your hearing loss

One would think that the more severe the deafness, the more likely is the person to feel trapped in a lonely world. Experts believe, though, that today's individuals with severe hearing loss and profound deafness are more likely to make better adjustments than those with mild and moderate hearing loss. Deaf people don't have to struggle to join in conversations, to hear music and so on; they are presented with a fait accompli, so generally do their utmost to live their lives to the full. Because they are likely to have developed hearing problems very early in life, they will have attended schools and social centres for the deaf and so have become part of a strong social group who share the same disability. They are also more likely to learn to lipread and use sign language, so can actually communicate very well within their social group.

People with mild and moderate hearing loss, on the other hand, still try to get by in a hearing world, with hearing people. If your hearing has diminished gradually with age, you have spent most of your life being able to communicate effectively with others and able to be spontaneous. To have these things removed and be cast into loneliness is very difficult. And when you find the people around you carelessly disregarding you, forgetting all about your hearing problem or even that you exist, it is nothing less than a nightmare. Many people with hearing loss admit to spending a lot of their time 'feeling like a fool', and react by withdrawing further from public gatherings.

Profound deafness

Until recent years, people with profound deafness were treated with superstition and judged as psychologically unbalanced, inferior human beings. In many ancient civilizations, deaf newborn babies were even thrown over a cliff or into deep water. When, in later years, the respected Greek philosopher Aristotle stated, among other things, that there was little point trying to communicate with deaf people, further negative feeling was engendered and spread down through the generations. Even today, the word 'dumb' is used by some people to describe someone inept, who acts without due thought of the consequences.

It is only within the last few hundred years that the many social and medical implications of deafness have begun to be researched by capable minds. However, there remains a great deal of prejudice and ignorance about profoundly deaf people and the hearing impaired. Indeed, they are still rejected from some schools, some college courses, some jobs, some societies and some social groups.

My opinion is that because people with normal hearing find it difficult to communicate with those who are hard of hearing – indeed, they often have to repeat themselves and make extra effort to speak up – they are prone to becoming annoyed and impatient. Of course, this often translates to a person with hearing loss, and can make them even less keen to join in.

Those who are born deaf would appear to suffer fewer knocks to their self-esteem than those who lose their hearing gradually. It's true that people with profound deafness can encounter a whole gamut of negative reactions from others when they try to enter a normal hearing environment; they are likely to need an interpreter when dealing with officials and so on, but for the most part they stick to their comfortable peer group and offer each other a great deal of support and encouragement. Most learn very early on to make the best of their inheritance, to enjoy their lives regardless. People with profound deafness are often given extra support in the work environment too, unlike those who develop gradual hearing loss and tend to struggle on alone, maybe attempting to hide the extent of their disability so they don't lose their job.

It is estimated that the profoundly deaf outnumber people with age-related hearing loss by 150 to 1.

Group situations

It is common for a person with hearing loss to be unsure of how to feel and behave when they're being ignored in a group situation.

Would it be best to guess at what's being said and add a comment of your own? But what if you repeat something that's already been said? What if your guess is wrong and your comment wildly out of place? Could you bear it if everyone laughed at you? Would you feel so humiliated you'd swear never again to try to join in? Alternatively, should you just shrink into yourself, allowing others to act as though you're not there? Or should you pretend – most of all to yourself – that you don't mind being ignored?

For many people, the sad thing about losing their hearing is that their personality undergoes a complete change. For example, Peter was a confident, inspirational web developer until hearing loss shattered his self-belief and made him feel 'apart' from the rest of his team. To his colleagues he became serious and formidable, and was no longer interested in either advancing his career or other people's lives. Tessa was once good-humoured, gregarious and the life and soul of the party, only to become introverted and irritable when she could no longer enjoy group situations. She began snapping at her husband and sons when they tried to encourage her to go out, and they found her sullen and difficult to please. It goes almost without saying that both Peter and Tessa are depressed and getting little from their lives.

It has been said that people who become hard of hearing actually suffer from paralysis of the personality. Just as someone who is physically paralysed can no longer step confidently into his or her former world, so a person with acquired hearing loss can no longer step confidently into a normal hearing environment. Even those who have learned to lipread find group situations very difficult. In meetings, for instance, they must stop volunteering to take the minutes; they are unable even to take notes for themselves as their eyes must at all times to be following the speaker's lips. When several people are speaking alternately, it is often not immediately evident who is now speaking and the gist of their dialogue can be lost in the time it takes to start reading their lips. A good friend of mine with hearing loss, Joann, told me she had tried to put forward a point of her own in a work meeting a few years back, only to be laughed at and told the point had already been made. She had missed it completely in the rapidity of orations and had vowed never again to attempt to join in. More fundamentally, however, the lipreader finds group situations intensely anxiety- and stress-provoking, not to mention mentally exhausting, for their eyes can never leave the speaker's lips, and their minds can't wander for a second. If they do wander, it can take some time to pick up the threads.

Many people with hearing loss have once enjoyed attending the theatre, the movies, shows and concerts, but can no longer follow the plot of the former two and can no longer fully appreciate the music in the latter two. And so, with reluctance, they stop going. People with profound deafness, it's sad to say, have never known the delights of such productions and may even be used to enjoying sign language plays.

The trauma of losing your hearing

It can take a while to realize you are losing your hearing, and once you do, it's a shock to your entire being. Not only do you imagine that your life will never be the same, but you also wonder if, in your new vulnerable state, you can survive in a world that relies so heavily on communication. Until we start to lose it, we all tend to take our hearing for granted, unaware of the many ways in which it functions throughout the day. We even rely on our hearing to wake us when we're sleeping (via an alarm clock), or when something is wrong (such as a burglar in the house or the baby crying). Once the ability to hear clearly has gone, we miss it more than we could ever have imagined, and more than it's possible to express to others. We feel angry, alone, frustrated, frightened, depressed and vulnerable – not to mention foolish when we misunderstand, and stupid when someone says loudly, 'Did you hear that?' or 'He's a bit deaf, you know!'

It often takes several years for a person who once had normal hearing to adjust to being hearing impaired. The inability to hear clearly, whether it has occurred over a short or long period, can create trauma that's not easy to overcome – after all, you have been robbed of your ability to cope with life, not to mention many of your dreams and aspirations for your future. That trauma, in those who have experienced gradual hearing loss, might not have been so great had they been prepared beforehand to cope with the psychological effects of being unable to hear properly. It's an unfortunate fact, though, that specialists in the hearing field still tend to concentrate on the practicalities, such as the use of hearing aids and sound amplification devices. You may be offered six to ten sessions of hearing therapy, but realistically, that's not nearly enough. Moreover, research into hearing loss does not constitute a priority for the government of today. We can only hope that the situation is about to change with the recent formation of the All-Party Parliamentary Group on Deafness.

Becoming hard of hearing instils many difficult emotions in the person concerned. However, it's necessary to go through many emotional stages before you can be ready to deal with your hearing shortfall.

Fear

After a strong sense of isolation, which is discussed throughout this book, comes the feeling of fear. The things commonly feared include the following:

- fear of new situations;
- fear of people;
- fear of group situations;
- fear of being ridiculed;
- fear of being snubbed;
- fear of being avoided;
- fear of being made conspicuous;
- fear of failure;
- fear of chance encounters;
- fear of sudden noises.

Coming to terms with hearing loss

Almost everyone who loses their good health or who suffers a sensory impairment such as hearing loss, goes through the same stages of denial, projection, anger, depression and finally acceptance. These stages are discussed below.

Denial

Because a very real threat to your physical and emotional wellbeing is difficult to accept, you are likely to experience denial in the early days of your hearing loss. Denial is particularly common when hearing loss has crept up on you slowly; it gives your emotions time to accept the new situation. Unfortunately, however, while in the grip of denial a person tries to carry on as before, making no attempt to adjust their lives to take account of their problem. In some people, denial is taken to the extreme. Lucy, for example, is accused by Bill, her husband, of not trying to understand the discussions at a neighbourhood watch meeting. When she replies, 'I didn't listen on purpose. Those people talk a lot of nonsense', Bill may get angry, feeling that Lucy is judging their neighbours unfairly. Further similar episodes can even provoke arguments between the couple.

However, there invariably comes a point when the individual has no choice but to acknowledge that there is a problem. In many cases, the problem is pointed out by family members who are frustrated by the continual excuses and finally realize what is going on.

Projection

Often, the next defence mechanism in the adjustment process is blaming the problem on someone else – a stage termed *projection*. Examples of projection are when Margaret repeatedly says to Claire, her daughter, 'Speak up! You do tend to mumble, you know!' After visiting a relative, she complains to Claire, 'I bet no one heard our Ruth properly – she had her stereo turned up loud when we were trying to talk' and, after a coffee in a shopping centre, 'I could hardly hear a word you said, Claire. The acoustics in that place were terrible.'

People with hearing loss often complain that the younger generation mutter incoherently, making them impossible to under-stand. It's true that elocution is rarely taught in schools these days and that young people do tend to mutter more than they did, but hearing people rarely complain of not understanding them – or at least not nearly so much as people who are hearing impaired.

Anger

As the individual begins to acknowledge that he or she does indeed have a problem, anger is liable to flare up at any time. Some people feel angry and resentful toward anything and everything. For instance, Stephen regularly makes comments such as, 'I can't believe it, it's raining again! That's another gardening day ruined!' and 'I'm not answering that phone any more. I've got better things to do!'

Other people direct their anger toward a particular person – usually their nearest and dearest. For instance, Michael often speaks to his wife, Josie, in the following way: 'I know you're ashamed of me when we go out together, so go out on your own in future!' and 'Can't you cook something I actually might like! I'm sick of your bland meals!' Although much of this anger is no doubt unwarranted, it's also important that the partner or carer avoid insensitive comments. Josie saying, 'You really embarrassed me when you didn't answer that question they asked. You started spouting on about something completely different', or 'Why don't you listen more carefully? You wouldn't miss so much then' will surely provoke a further angry outburst that could have been avoided.

Depression

When all anger is spent, sinking into depression is generally the next stage. This is reactive depression, caused by something specific – the loss of the ability to hear well. It's at this point that individuals often start to distance themselves from social situations and retreat into themselves. An abrupt personality change may also occur – for instance, the person may become sullen and self-centred. As a result, family and friends are liable to feel nervous and even afraid of the new person in their midst, which makes the individual feel more isolated than ever.

At this stage, people with hearing loss become acutely aware of their vulnerability. They can no longer hear someone creeping up on them from behind, tampering with the door or moving about downstairs at night. Also, it now dawns on them fully that life as they knew it has drawn to a close and that it will be a struggle from now on. It doesn't help that the absence of background noise such as birds singing, rain falling, wind blowing and tap-water trickling gives rise to a 'dead' feeling, which is now fully absorbed.

The depression of hearing loss is short-lived in some people, but can last for many years in others. It depends on the character of the person concerned.

Acceptance

Again depending on the character of the person concerned, it can take weeks, months or even many years to travel through the different stages of grieving until acceptance – defined in my dictionary as the willingness to tolerate a difficult or unpleasant situation – is reached. Acceptance can only come after depression has lifted, and involves the realization that you don't want to miss out on things any more.

It is only when you are resigned to being hearing impaired that psychological counselling can be effective. Also, it's at this point that you may want to try using a hearing aid (see Chapter 6 for information on how to use a hearing aid properly). If you attempt to use a hearing aid before fully accepting your hearing disability, you are likely not to give it a proper trial. Hearing aids require a lot of time and patience, as well as motivation. Your emotions should be stabilized to give a hearing aid the best chance.

Overcompensation

As the psychiatrist P. H. Knapp found on working with men who became deaf during World War II, there are some who travel through additional stages before reaching acceptance. One such stage is overcompensation, where the person adopts an extrovert attitude, talking incessantly to anyone who'll listen. In so doing, he or she avoids the need for speechreading and understanding the other person.

Exploitation

Some individuals with hearing loss make it crystal clear to the people around them that they are now invalids. Indeed, they use the status of invalidism to gain sympathy from others and actually to exploit their feelings of compassion and concern. For instance, Victor is now having his wife running up and down the stairs to get things for him, filling in forms because he 'doesn't feel up to it', and taking over the driving because he's 'stressed enough and can't cope with any more'.

The victim

It is not unusual for people with hearing loss to cast themselves in the role of victim. This takes the form of withdrawing from society and feeling discriminated against. Of course, people who have locked themselves behind closed doors for a length of time can find enforced communication supremely difficult. It's not always possible to get out of talking to other people, and it is always more difficult to communicate when you are out of the habit of doing so and have not learned ways and means of helping yourself.

Getting stuck at one stage

You can tell whether you have been stuck at one stage for too long by looking at whether the characteristics of a particular stage are damaging your lifestyle, personality and relationships with others. If you can see that your emotions are controlling you and causing harm to your life, you would be best advised to seek the help of an audiologist or hearing therapist. First, though, you may wish to attempt to work out your own problems, which you may be able to do with the help of this book. You can start by telling yourself that your hearing will not be restored, and that you will get more from your life if you can accept this fact. Actively seeking ways to overcome your communication problems can move you ahead more quickly, for it enables you to see that you can still feel a part of things.

Developing a healthy attitude

To help yourself and the people around you, it is essential that you feel better about your hearing problem. Taking heed of the following pointers will help you to develop a more positive attitude:

- Your hearing loss affects other people. Be prepared to deal with their reactions, whatever they may be (see Chapter 4).

- Find out as much as you can about the physical and psychological effects of hearing loss. Really try to absorb all the ways you can improve your communication skills.
- Recognize when you are using emotional factors as an excuse. For instance, if you are taking out your anger on your partner, be aware of that fact and endeavour to alter it. Your husband may think you are truly angry with him, rather than with your problem. If you tend to accuse other people of mumbling, recognize that fact and acknowledge that it's really you who have the problem, not them. It's important that you accept responsibility instead of passing it on to an innocent party. If you can get into the habit of analysing your feelings, you will make great progress.
- Admit to the people around you that you have a hearing problem and explain that they can help you by speaking more clearly, facing you when speaking and so on.
- Be willing to accept help from others – feeling patronized is counterproductive. You have a communication problem and need to accept assistance to be able to take part effectively in conversations.
- Accept that your hearing impairment is your responsibility. Don't expect other people to solve the problem, and avoid taking out your frustrations on them.

When the people around you see that you are trying to help yourself, they will invariably react favourably, attempting to help you to improve even more. These factors will be discussed in more detail throughout this book.

When a family member has hearing loss

Virtually everyone in the developed world lives or works with someone with hearing loss, or has a relative, friend or acquaintance who suffers from it. Many people know at least a handful of individuals who are hearing impaired, making it appear like a natural part of life that has to be endured. Relatives may therefore fail to find practical help and emotional support for an affected family member. This problem is then compounded by the lack of easily accessible information about what can be done to aid communication. It's unfortunate, too, that numerous doctors still tell their patients that nothing can be done to improve their condition and that they will just have to live with it.

4

Coping strategies

Communication difficulties are the great bane of life for people with hearing loss. Fortunately, there are a number of coping strategies that can be of terrific help. If you can put these strategies into practice, you will be more able to socialize and deal with the practicalities of life, such as shopping, speaking to the plumber, having your car serviced and so on. As a result, you will suffer far less anxiety and stress and be able to get on with your life.

An American psychologist, Samuel Trychin, who has himself been hard of hearing for many years, has devised these strategies. Dr Trychin has written a series of books and articles on coping with hearing loss, and conducts workshops and training programmes across the USA and in Canada.

Understand your particular hearing problem

You can help yourself, first of all, by knowing as much as possible about your particular hearing problem. When you see your audiologist, ask for an interpretation of your audiogram – the graphic record produced by your hearing tests. The audiologist will be able to show you where your hearing loss lies with regard to the 'speech banana' – a statistical representation of speech sounds. The speech banana is not an easy concept to grasp, so if you fail to understand what you're being told, don't be afraid to ask the audiologist to go through it again.

The audiogram measures your hearing threshold at each frequency of sound. When you look at your particular audiogram – with the help of your audiologist – it may be apparent that you can hear more of the lower frequency speech sounds than the higher ones, or vice versa. A person who can hear mainly the lower frequency speech sounds will have problems with the high frequencies where consonants have their predominant energy. For example, the sounds *f, s, t, v, ch, sh, th, k, z,* and *p* will be difficult to hear or be mostly unheard, and consonants contribute more to the understanding of speech than anything else. A person with high frequency loss will primarily hear low frequency vowels and soft-voiced consonants, which may not make a lot of sense. Every case is different and you really need your audiologist to spell out which parts of speech you are finding it difficult to pick up.

It is also recommended that you ask the audiologist which environmental sounds you will have difficulty hearing – for example, a baby crying, the doorbell and telephone ringing, a dog barking, a smoke alarm bleeping, a police or ambulance siren blaring. You then should inform your friends and family members of your hearing problem areas. Their understanding can help them to avoid misinterpreting your failure to hear some sounds, therefore avoiding arguments, hurt feelings and damaged relationships.

Do I speak too loudly or too quietly?

It is common for a person with hearing loss sometimes to speak more loudly than necessary, and at other times not loudly enough. Speaking too loudly results from wanting to hear yourself more clearly. On the other hand, when there is background noise that your ears are not picking up very well, you may not realize you need to raise your voice above it.

To judge how to pitch your voice, it's advisable that you assess each particular situation. You will soon become adept at gauging how best to pitch your voice. The factors to take into consideration are as follows:

- If the person you are conversing with winces slightly or backs away a little when you speak, it's safe to say you can lower your voice.
- If the other person leans nearer to you as you speak, he or she may not be hearing you clearly and you should try raising your voice.
- If there is obvious background noise, such as in a shopping centre or a busy street, you would be best raising your voice. This

also applies if there is a fan blowing in the room, the TV is turned on or there is a nearby open window with traffic outside.

Don't be afraid to ask friends and family whether your voice is pitched at the right level. This should also have the effect of making others more aware that they need to speak up, speak more clearly and so on.x

Communication problem areas

Research has shown that when a person with impaired hearing fails to understand what someone is saying, he or she is likely to blame their hearing disability. The truth is, however, that many factors can add to communication problems, and it's not always your fault – not by any means. If these problems are recognized for what they are, you can then try to resolve the difficulty and improve your understanding.

Common causes of communication breakdown are speaker factors, environmental factors and listener factors, all of which are discussed below.

Speaker factors

These factors include the way the other person speaks, i.e. the speed, loudness and clarity. Your understanding of speech can also be affected by facial hair, distracting mannerisms, a distorted public address system, a foreign accent or a strong regional dialect. Of course, whether the person is facing you at the time of speaking is another factor, as is how close you are to the speaker.

Also, it is not always possible, when you are with several people, to see everyone's mouths. You can overcome this by arriving early at venues so you can choose the seat from which you have the best range of visibility. If your problem is a distorted public address system, don't be afraid to ask the person nearest to you what was announced. That way you know on which platform to catch your train, whether it's your turn to go in to see the doctor, and whether it's your car that's blocking an entrance.

When the other person has facial hair, a foreign accent or regional dialect, you can do little but try to concentrate more intently on what they are saying. However, if the other person is speaking too quickly, too quietly, mumbling or waving their arms about, it's recommended that you calmly explain that you have a hearing problem and politely ask them to slow down, speak up, speak more clearly or try to stop waving their arms about.

Repeatedly saying, 'Eh?' or 'What?' can be very annoying – even exasperating. It can give the impression that you're not really paying attention. In this case, after explaining that you are hard of hearing, try to be creative in the way you ask for a repeat. For example, 'I didn't catch that last bit …' means they only need repeat the last few words. A good trick, if you're not sure you heard properly, is to use the information you did catch to phrase your question – i.e. 'What time did you say you'd be arriving?' 'What was that about Philip?' and 'Your appointment is on Thursday, is that right?'

By altering the level and speed of your own voice, it is sometimes possible to change the way other people speak. For example, a soft voice can encourage a soft response and speaking more slowly can prompt the other person to speak more slowly. Your demeanour can also affect the way others respond to you. Hanging back and trying not to be noticed can make people either ignore you, or speak to you half-heartedly. However, holding yourself with confidence and looking directly at the other person encourages them to respond in a full and clear voice.

Environmental factors

Environmental factors that can impede understanding include background noise, poor lighting, visual or auditory distractions, obstacles that impede your view, poor ventilation and absence of assistive listening devices.

You can try to counter these things by either moving closer to the speaker, asking them politely to stop smoking for a while so you can see their lips moving or to move so the light hits them better, or by explaining your hearing problem and asking if he or she would mind accompanying you to a place you know to be more listener-friendly (the next room, for example). Background noise is the great bugbear of the hearing impaired, and the easiest ways to deal with it are either to choose your location or change the situation. For instance, in a restaurant, it's best to ask for a table away from the kitchen, the instrumentalists or any other noisy spot. At home, don't forget to turn off the television, radio or stereo system when you are trying to communicate with someone.

Listener factors

Factors that can prevent the listener from understanding conversation include the type and severity of their hearing loss, their ability to concentrate, motivation to hear, levels of tiredness and tension and their emotional state. Getting into the habit of assessing the situation for barriers to communication and learning how to reduce their effects will enable conversations to be more easily understood.

If you wear a hearing aid, don't forget that it may not be functioning correctly and so may be causing you additional problems. Or you may simply keep forgetting to turn it on. A faulty hearing aid should be returned to your audiologist, who will repair it as soon as possible. You may own a hearing aid, but never felt it worked for you properly, in which case your audiologist can advise you on developing proper listening skills. Those of you who have never used a hearing aid, yet struggle to hear every word said, would be best advised to ask for a referral to an audiologist with a view to getting one (see Chapter 6 for more information on hearing aids).

Because for the hard of hearing lipreading is such a large part of understanding, having poor eyesight is an obvious disadvantage. However, it's your responsibility to have your eyesight checked regularly and to wear the most appropriate glasses you can. There may also be times when you are just not motivated to listen, especially if the conversation is not stimulating enough. As a result, the attention you normally give to listening will falter and concentration levels fall. You should try to recognize when you are 'tuning out' due to lack of interest, and not blame this on your problems with hearing. People with hearing loss will tend to 'tune out' more than hearing people without realizing it. This is because hearing is much more of an effort and it's easy to stop focusing when the subject doesn't grab you.

Here are a few pointers to make listening easier:

- Take a moment to pause and think about what you have heard. This can enable you to fill in the blanks and so work out what you missed.
- When you are asking a question of someone, try to be specific. Asking 'Does this bus go past Beamish Avenue?' will bring a direct yes or no answer, whereas a more general question, such as 'Where does this bus stop?' can bring a more complex response that is more difficult to follow.
- Instead of continually trying to follow conversations, try introducing a topic of your own. It is easier to be a part of a conversation when you are familiar with the topic and many of the relevant words. However, be careful not to introduce the same topics repeatedly – this can be tiresome for other people. Moreover, don't be tempted to do all the talking just because it's easier than listening.
- Don't worry about catching every word spoken. Many people with hearing loss are bothered by every word they miss and desperately wish they could catch everything. This only makes them stressed and anxious, which is counterproductive.
- When you are asking for instructions or directions, for example, it is best to ask the other person to write them down so that there is no confusion. This is particularly important for instructions on taking medications.
- In meetings, ask the chairperson to ensure that people don't talk over each other. Other people are likely to appreciate this as well. Making sure you have a copy of the agenda will help you to know what topic is coming up next.
- When a remark you make is clearly out of context, you may worry about what other people think of you. Try not to waste energy on negative emotions! Do your best to laugh it off and remind yourself of the many times you get it right. Adopting a positive mental attitude and good sense of humour works wonders. It might start off as forced, but with time, positivity and good humour can become your natural mind-set.

Decide what you want to listen to

It's a natural tendency to want to hear most of what's going on around you, but even people with normal hearing can only absorb one conversation at a time. If close to a competing noise, a person with hearing loss has no hope at all of hearing everything around them. Instead they often struggle to follow just one conversation.

Upon entering a difficult listening situation, make a conscious decision about whom or what you plan to listen to. For instance, at a concert, you may prefer to concentrate on the music, rather than worrying about also hearing the comments of your companion. In a bar, you will probably choose to listen only to your two friends rather than the conversations around you, or the background music. Making such decisions can relieve a lot of stress and anxiety and help you to tune in to your preferred sounds.

Informing others of your hearing problem

To overcome each of the above types of problem, it's essential that you inform the other person of your problems with hearing. Explaining politely, in a matter-of-fact way – taking some of the blame yourself – should have the effect of the other person wanting to help you to understand. If other people are not aware of your hearing impairment, there is a high risk that any inappropriate replies you make will be attributed to something unfavourable. For example, people with hearing loss can be thought of as stupid, confused, aloof, weird, unfriendly, inept, lazy, not interested and so on, when in fact they simply misunderstand what is being said or don't realize they are being spoken to.

Communication breakdown is always a risk for someone with hearing loss, but if you can inform the other person that your hearing isn't what it was, you avoid being unfairly condemned. However, once you have explained your problem, it's important that you also politely inform the other person of what he or she can do to help you understand. Simply saying, 'What?' 'Pardon?' 'I'm sorry, I didn't catch that', 'Would you repeat that?' when you fail to understand something will not necessarily alert the other person to the fact that you are hard of hearing, neither does it inform them of what to do to improve communication between you. After you have explained your hearing problem, it is probably best to say something like, 'So, if you don't mind, you can help me by slowing down a little', or 'I need to see your lips moving – I try to speechread, you see. So would you mind please speaking as clearly as you can and looking at me at the same time?' or 'Because of my hearing problems, would you mind speaking up a bit more?'

When asked to change their behaviour, some people may feel criticized and react by becoming defensive. It's therefore important that you put the onus on yourself. Saying 'Because of my hearing problems ...' prior to asking them to do something different avoids them feeling criticized.

If a foreign accent is the problem, you obviously can't ask the other person to get rid of it. All you can do here is be aware that your inability to understand some of the things said isn't all your fault.

In some cases, the content of what is said may be a problem in itself. For example, when a piece of news, information, an instruction, message, lecture and so on is long-winded, detailed and perhaps boring, it will be far more difficult to understand – see 'Listener factors' in the previous section. It may be possible to prepare in advance, finding a book or internet site from which you can swot up the subject. However, you may have no choice but to accept that certain dialogues will always be out of your scope.

Reminding others of your problem

If you have previously explained your hearing loss to a particular person, it doesn't harm to say, 'Because of my hearing problems ...' by way of reminding them that you have difficulties hearing and that they need to adjust their manner of speaking.

Try not to feel annoyed or dismayed when others immediately forget what you asked them to do. It's a fact that we are all more interested in what we are saying than how we are saying it. We get caught up in the moment and can think only of passing on a particular piece of information, advice or gossip. Moreover, it's far from easy to change habitual unconscious behaviour of any kind, and each of us has been speaking in a particular manner for as far back as we can remember.

When anticipating different behaviour from others, you need a great deal of patience. They will no doubt continually forget to do as you ask, and you may feel angry and frustrated, which gets you nowhere. Unfortunately, repeatedly asking the other person to speak more slowly and so on can become irritating to both parties – it is therefore recommended that you use certain gestures to serve as a reminder. Hand gestures are particularly useful as they avoid the need to keep verbally interrupting. Here are some examples:

- raising the palm of a hand a little can be the reminder to speak up;
- a hand with the palm facing down moved in a downward motion can be the reminder to speak more slowly;
- a finger turning anti-clockwise can be the signal for the speaker to repeat what they just said;
- making exaggerated lip movements as you speak can be the reminder to the other person to speak more clearly.

A useful communication strategy is to model the behaviour you would like from others. For example, if you would like your partner and family members to stop talking to you from another room, you should avoid doing that yourself. If you would like them to stop speaking to you in unnaturally raised voices, you should try to moderate your own tone so it is at the level you would like others to use. If you would like others to stop speaking so quickly, you should speak at the rate you prefer to hear.

These strategies don't always work, but they're still worth trying. You never know: most of your family and friends might pick up on them very quickly. There will always be people who are so set in their behaviour that you may have to point out that you would appreciate them speaking to you in a particular manner. If you make polite requests rather than demands, others are far more likely to comply.

Be wary of making negative responses

When a problem arises in communication, both the speaker and listener will react in some way. A positive reaction on your part should resolve the problem, whereas a negative one will make the situation worse and bode badly for future communication with that person. For example, if you try to bluff your way through, withdraw from the conversation or dominate it on a regular basis, you are likely to become angry, frustrated, anxious and depressed.

It's always helpful if you can learn to pause to identify the cause of the problem. For example, it may be that there is too much background noise or that you need the other person to move their hands from their mouth. Telling the person that you would hear better if you sat at a distance from the music speakers or that you would be able to speechread more easily if they would very kindly move their hands away from their mouth are constructive reactions and will normally gain a positive response. Making a conscious decision to relax with others will also help. Being tense and anxious only serves to make communication more difficult than it need be.

Not understanding

Friends and family members of a person with hearing loss may often complain that they're never sure when you have understood and when you have misunderstood. And not knowing can be frustrating and annoying. The only way to avoid this is to acknowledge in some way that you haven't understood what was said, and to offer a suggestion for resolving the problem. You could use the signals mentioned earlier, such as a finger turning anti-clockwise so the speaker knows to repeat what they said, or the palm of the hand raised so the speaker knows to raise the volume a little. Showing the speaker appreciation for having the patience to go through things again is vital too. If you omit to thank them – it need take only a smile and quick nod of the head – you risk having your requests for co-operation met with irritation and annoyance.

Misunderstanding

A very common problem for someone with hearing loss is misunderstanding what was said. Of course, although they might not know it, this is also a problem for the other person for it signals a communication breakdown. Janice, for example, thought she heard her husband, Keith, say, 'I'm going to re-book that holiday', which confused Janice as she'd believed they were both excited about their up-coming holiday. It soon emerged, however, that what Keith had actually said was, 'I'm going to read a book on that holiday.' In the same way, Cathy thought her friend Megan had said, 'Would you like me to take some cones for the party?' When Cathy's reply was a bewildered, 'Why would we want traffic cones at the party?' Megan realized the misunderstanding and repeated, 'I said, would you like me to bake some scones for the party?'

The occasional misunderstanding can be quite funny, but when it happens numerous times throughout the day – as it frequently does with hearing loss in the equation – both parties can become exasperated and weary. The consequences can be devastating in relationships, especially where appointment times, places to meet, people's names and so on are concerned. In the workplace, when instructions, figures, account details and other important information are misunderstood, the consequences can be serious.

It is not helped when the person who is hard of hearing indicates that they have understood, for there's every chance that they have misunderstood completely. The best step for the person with the hearing problem is actually to repeat the important detail, such as the name, phone number, time, location and date. For example, saying 'You said Tuesday morning at eleven o'clock, outside Shipley town hall' can highlight the fact that the location is actually Chigley, not Shipley. Following the advice under 'Listener factors' above should also prove helpful.

Putting the strategies into practice

It's plain to see that once you start employing the above strategies, they should facilitate easier communication. However, the strategies need using many times to come easily and feel natural. The early days of putting them into practice are the most difficult, and it's best to get used to applying them at home with enlightened family members before putting yourself under pressure to use them when you're out and about. If they can become second nature at home, you should automatically start using them more with other people.

Still far too many hearing-impaired people are oblivious to the fact that there is help available – this also applies to their families and carers. There are several books that discuss coping strategies and help you to deal with the common problems related to hearing loss (see the Further Reading section at the back of this book). There are also local and national resources for the hard of hearing, including counselling and psychological support. My advice is to take all the help you are offered, and if you feel you need to, actively seek more.

Being assertive

It is said that the most valuable attribute a person with hearing loss can develop is assertiveness. Standing up for your rights – but in the process avoiding hurting or irritating other people – helps to ensure that you communicate effectively most of the time. Assertiveness also helps you to feel good about yourself, unlike when you are continually passive and allow people to walk all over you, or frequently aggressive so you scare people off.

Passive behaviour

Unfortunately, there may be times when others try to take advantage of your hearing loss, in which case speaking up for yourself can halt them in their tracks. For instance, Sarah handled her hearing loss by nodding and smiling a lot, trying to hide the fact that she was hearing little of what was said. She would also avoid eye contact so no one would speak to her, stare blankly and pretend she wasn't interested, let someone else be her interpreter, and avoid more and more social situations. She felt bad about herself and reinforced her poor self-image by letting people ignore her, allowing people to keep her waiting and so on because they knew she wouldn't stand up for herself. Sarah was trapped in a vicious circle, becoming increasingly quiescent and subdued as time went by.

Aggressive behaviour

As mentioned, some people react to their hearing impairment by being angry and aggressive. For instance, Jack constantly blamed others for speaking too quietly; insisted he didn't have a problem; demanded that others help him; dominated the conversation so he didn't have to listen and became generally infuriated by his communication difficulties. Of course, people disliked the way he was behaving and took to avoiding him. Before long, Jack was feeling lonely and cut off. Although his ego was inflated due to his ability to get his own way, in truth he was the loser.

Assertive behaviour

Keeping calm, standing up for your rights and generally taking the middle ground can pay dividends. For instance, Connie had learned through her job in management that she could get more from her staff when she expressed herself appropriately, valuing her own rights as well as those of her staff. When she began losing her hearing, she used the same technique to ensure that she was able to communicate. For example, she was proactive in saying, 'Sorry, but my hearing's not as sharp as it was. Can you speak up a bit, please?' She was taking responsibility for her problem and politely asking the other person to help. As a result, Connie hung on to her self-respect and that of most of the people around her – and that made her feel good about herself. It's therefore very important for people with hearing loss to be assertive.

5

A hearing therapy programme

The three most important methods of understanding speech are hearing, seeing and life experiences. The first part of this chapter will concentrate on these, and the second part will focus on blending what you have learned into speechreading, which simply means having the ability to use hearing, seeing and life experiences to work out what is being said when the words are not heard completely.

As speechreading depends largely on being able to lipread, it's recommended that you join your nearest lipreading class. Here, you will not only be taught the intricacies of lipreading, you will also be able to practise the technique as much as you like. You will meet lots of people in the same situation as yourself, too, and should find it a friendly, supportive environment.

All the aspects of this chapter will be of more benefit to you if used in conjunction with professional guidance – from an audiologist or other hearing specialist, such as a speech–language pathologist.

Hearing

Individuals with normal hearing must generally make an effort to *tune out* background noise and other noises around them. However, people with hearing loss need to *tune in* actively to the sounds they want to hear – background noise is a great problem, as is being spoken to in a very soft voice. As mentioned earlier, you need to make a conscious decision about whom or what you want to listen to, moving to a quieter location if necessary and ensuring there's enough light for you to see the other person clearly.

The following suggestions may also help:

- Think hard about the subject being discussed so that you are partly prepared for the words and phrases to come.
- Stare at the speaker's lips to make maximum use of your lipreading ability. The more you try to lipread, the quicker you will improve. Lipreading also helps to focus your attention.
- Consider the direction the sound you are trying to listen to is coming from. If the speaker is at your side, move so that you are facing them.
- Consider the distance between yourself and the speaker. Move closer if necessary.
- In your home, move your seating so that you are directly facing your guests. Ensure the other seating is not too distant from your own chair.

Seeing

With training and practice, it is possible for a person with hearing loss to recognize more than just the obvious mouth movements – but it's a myth that good lipreaders can easily follow a conversation. The truth is, there will always be words they misread or fail to catch altogether. In fact, 70 per cent of sounds in the English language look very much alike on the lips, such as *b*, *p* and *m*. Without hearing the word or working it out from context, it's impossible to differentiate between the words 'bat', 'pat' and 'mat', for all are made with the lips pressed together.

Lipreading is also handicapped by the average speed at which we speak. Indeed, the eye and brain are only able to process eight or nine mouth movements a second, while 13 mouth movements a second are made in normal speech. Even if the correct words are deciphered, the lipreader will always be trailing the speaker and may often fall so far behind that anxiety takes over and the thread of the conversation is lost. It doesn't help that some people fail to move their mouths very much during speech. Moreover, neighbouring sounds affect the way a sound looks on the lips. For example, note the shape of your mouth when you say the different words 'bee' and 'bow'.

All in all, lipreading is not the whole answer for a person who is hard of hearing. It can provide valuable clues to the gist of the conversation, especially when assessed in conjunction with facial expressions and bodily movements. These things are often ignored but are essential parts of the process of speechreading.

Speechreading

The speechreading technique is a supplement to lipreading and involves several factors, including lipreading, looking at body language and facial expressions, and being aware of the five basic groups of sounds that are visible on the lips. These sounds are as follows:

- *B*, *p* and *m* – made with the lips pressed together.
- *Th* (pronounced as in either 'theatre' or 'there') – formed with the lips parted and the tongue slightly protruding or behind the top teeth.
- *F* and *v* – made by bringing the upper teeth in contact with the bottom lip. The top lip does not touch the bottom lip, unlike with *b*, *p*, and *m*.
- *W* and *r* – produced by a rounding of the lips. You can differentiate between the two by observing the slight protrusion of the lips in the *w*.
- *Sh*, *ch* and sounds like *j* as in 'jet' and *y* as in 'young' – formed by a rounding and definite protrusion of the lips. The lips open more for these sounds than for *w* and *r*.

To speechread effectively, it is important to commit to memory the lip movements for the above five groups of sounds. This is best achieved by watching yourself speak in a mirror. In time, you will recognize to which group of sounds a particular lip movement belongs – automatically and without effort. Unfortunately, other sounds such as *g*, *n* and *k* are formed in the mouth and not on the lips, so are not easy to distinguish. Moreover, the vowel sounds (*a*, *e*, *i*, *o*, *u*) are so influenced by the consonants around them that recognition is difficult. Vowels are generally spoken more loudly, however, and you may be able to hear them more clearly.

In learning to identify the basic groups, practise lipreading with a partner using normal conversation and carry out the exercises given later in this chapter. It isn't good enough for your partner to just mouth certain words, for they are formed differently in the mouth when spoken aloud. Also, please note that the art of speechreading must be learned phonetically, and you should get used to seeing how it looks on the lips. Forget how the word is spelled – that's of no consequence at all. With practice and constant awareness of visual clues, you should eventually be able to follow most conversations.

The following are examples of visual clues given by the speaker:

- A shrug and a quick glance at the clock should help you to understand: 'I don't know what time I'm supposed to be meeting Rachel.'
- A shake of the head should help you to understand: 'Today's gone so fast.'
- Raised outstretched palms will help you to understand: 'Who knows? He's a law unto himself.'
- A hand pressed to the stomach can help you to understand: 'I had an awful stomach ache last night.'
- Puffed-out cheeks can help you to understand: 'I'm feeling really bored/exhausted.'

Life experience

Your life experience – your grasp of the English language and under-standing of various situations – is likely to be the most important tool you have in the speechreading process. Indeed, it can be seen from the examples given below that you don't need to understand every word to know what is being said.

Conceptual closure

It is still difficult to be certain of what people are saying just by lipreading and looking for visual clues. Having an instinct for *what is likely to be said* in a particular situation can make all the difference to your understanding. For example, if you know the subject being discussed is last night's TV thriller, you are more likely to under-stand, 'I was surprised when he bound and gagged her.' You may not have been able to hear whether the speaker had said 'pound', 'bound' or 'mound', but within the context of the topic and the rest of the sentence, you are likely to work it out quickly. This process of filling in the blanks is called conceptual closure.

Grammatical closure

The mind can also work out what was said by means of a process termed grammatical closure, where knowledge of basic grammar helps to fill in the blanks. For example, if you hear something like, 'The dog are in the garden', it's clear from the word 'are' that there is more than one dog and therefore that the word must have been 'dogs'. This works the same way with the past tense. For example, if you hear, 'He work until late, yesterday', it's clear that the past tense is being used and that the word 'work' should really be 'worked'.

Getting confused

The important thing about conceptual and grammatical closure is to stop yourself getting hung up on trying to understand two or three words, and so miss the remainder of the sentence. Trying to follow the overall gist of the conversation is what is important. Also, it's vital to remember that people generally make sense when they talk. For example, don't tie yourself in knots trying to work out what your daughter meant by 'When we used to play Tommy Toes, I always cheated.' You have no recollection of playing a game called 'Tommy Toes'. So what other games have you played with your daughter – ones at which she cheated? The pair of you used to play dominoes when she was small, and you often let her win. So there you have the answer! She's talking about dominoes.

Knowing what to expect

In addition, you have a better chance of understanding conversation if you know what to expect. Much of everyday gossip is based on topics in the newspapers and magazines. It's advisable, therefore, to read a daily newspaper and a weekly magazine so that you are informed about current affairs, the latest movies, celebrity gossip and so on.

If the conversation takes a sudden turn, you should find it easier to join in if you quickly prepare yourself. For example, if holidays abroad are now being discussed, remind yourself of some words you might hear, such as 'flight', 'beach', 'hot', 'swimming', 'bars', 'hotel' and 'sunbathing'. Alternatively, if cars are being discussed, be prepared to hear the names of different car manufacturers and models, as well as the words 'gears', 'power-steering', 'air conditioning', 'central-locking', 'mileage', 'lead-free petrol' and 'suspension'. Now make a determined effort to recognize these words in conversation.

It's a good idea to invent a situation with a partner – such as booking a seat at the theatre, buying groceries from the corner shop and speaking to a plumber about a leak. You must first agree on the topic, then your partner should whisper several relevant words while you try to lipread. It will soon be clear how much easier it is to understand the words 'stop-tap', 'blocked' and 'flooded', for example, when they appear in context.

A similar exercise to improve your speechreading ability is to think of a variety of topics and mull over the related words you are likely to hear (see Exercise 3 in the following section). If you perform this exercise on a regular basis, you will learn to quickly predict the words you might hear.

Speechreading exercises

To enable you to maximize your speechreading skills, practise the following exercises as often as you can. Remember that it's not possible to lipread perfectly, and that there will always be words and phrases you are unable to recognize by eye.

It will invariably help if you are able to collect as much information as possible from gestures and facial expressions. Don't put yourself under pressure to work out every word said, however. Speechreading is barely more than a series of educated guesses and it's good enough to be aware of the gist of the conversation. Allow yourself to be content with that – and don't forget to congratulate yourself for being able to communicate fairly well when you don't always hear much of what's being said.

If you use a hearing aid, it should be turned on while most of the exercises given in this chapter are carried out.

Exercise 1

Watch a TV soap, drama or film with the sound muted and your hearing aid turned off. Try to work out the gist of the story and verbal exchanges by gestures and facial expressions alone.

Exercise 2

Without reading the print, look at pictures of people in newspapers and magazines and try to imagine their mood at the time the photo was taken. Do you think they are upset, angry, happy or puzzled? Is the person talking or listening? The more you try to work out a person's mood, the more accurate you should become.

Exercise 3

As already discussed, you will be more able to understand conversations if you prepare yourself for the words and phrases you might hear. Here are a few more examples:

Situation	Phrases you might expect to be said
Visiting your doctor	Try to describe the pain.
	Would you mind lying on the couch?
	Can you roll up your sleeve, please?
	I'm going to prescribe some tablets.
	How often has this happened?
In a shop	What can I do for you?
	Would you like help with packing these up?
	Do you remember what price this was?
	Would you like cash-back?
	Do you have something smaller?

Situation	Phrases you might expect to be said
At the hairdresser's	Do you just want a trim?
	Would you like a cut and blow dry?
	Have you been on holiday this year?
	Would you like a cup of coffee?
	Do you live nearby?

Exercise 4

This exercise should get you accustomed to the letters that can sound the same to a person with hearing loss. Ask a partner to say a random word from the groups below – adding more words to the groups if necessary. Rather than making a guess at the whole word and becoming frustrated because you keep getting it wrong, simply try to work out which group it is from. Your partner should say, first of all, whether you should be trying to identify the beginning or ending of a word. If you can tell that the word comes from the *ch* and *sh* group of endings, that's a great start! It's best to get used to working out which group of sounds a word belongs to before you go on to actually guessing the words in Exercise 5.

Words beginning with b, p *and* m *sounds:*

BAT	PUT	MAD	POLE	BALL	MADE
PAD	BEAD	MOUSE	BIN	PEAT	MORE

Words ending with b, p *and* m *sounds:*

HAM	BIB	LIP	SEEP	HOPE	SOME
SLAP	HIM	POPE	CHEAP	TAB	LAMB

Words beginning with f *and* v *sounds:*

FOUR	VAN	VEST	FORM	VINE	FOOT
FOAM	VAIN	FIVE	VILE	FAT	VEAL

Words ending with f *and* v *sounds:*

LIVE	SAVE	LAUGH	TIFF	LEAVE	SAFE
GRAPH	DIVE	HIVE	LEAF	SURF	ENOUGH

Words beginning with th *sounds:*
THORN   THREAD   THREE   THE   THAT   THING

Words ending with th *sounds:*
PATH   FAITH   TOOTH   WITH   BOOTH   MOUTH

Words beginning with w *and* r *sounds:*
WAIT   WHEAT   ROOT   WRITE   WARN   RING

Words ending with w *and* r *sounds:*
GNAW   LIAR   SLOW   RAW   HOW   CHEER

Words beginning with sh *and* ch *sounds:*
SHOW   CHEAT   SHAPE   CHAP   CHURN   SHINE

Words ending with sh *and* ch *sounds:*
LASH   INCH   BRANCH   DISH   LEASH   BIRCH

Exercise 5

After you've had a lot of practice at fitting words into groups of sounds, you can go on to the next stage – that of attempting to guess the word. When a partner whispers a word (not loud enough for you to hear it), think about which group it belongs in. You may want to see the word on the other person's lips a second time, but if you have already deduced that it begins with the sound *f* or *v*, watch really closely and try to see what it actually is.

This exercise is easier if your partner whispers similar sounding words – with the same vowel sounds, for example. Ask them to choose a set of three words from the groups below and try to work out each one in turn.

CAT	THAT	PLAIT
SUIT	FLUTE	ROOT
STAY	MAY	PLAY
WRITE	SIGHT	KITE
SEEM	DREAM	TEAM
BROWN	DROWN	FROWN

PINCH	FINCH	CINCH
DUE	FEW	QUEUE
RHYME	TIME	LIME
TALE	NAIL	VEIL
HEAT	WHEAT	BEAT
START	CART	HEART
MOLE	SOUL	ROLL

Exercise 6

When you feel you are getting the hang of recognizing endings, have your partner whisper words with the same beginnings. For now, stick to the same vowel sounds in each group of three. Using this principle, ask your partner to whisper other groups of words for you to decipher.

LOCK	LOT	LOB
BATCH	BAN	BAT
TIN	TIP	TICK
MOON	MOOSE	MOVE
HAY	HATE	HAIL

Exercise 7

Ask a partner to whisper each of the following sentences while you try to work out which group of sounds is used most in each. Using this principle, have your partner make up other phrases for you to decipher.

TESS TOOK A TRAY OF TARTS TO TOM
MY MOTHER MADE A MELON MOUSSE
LOOK AT THAT LADY LAUGHING OUT LOUD
THE CHAP CHEATED AT CHESS

Exercise 8

We looked at grammatical closure earlier in this chapter. Now, ask a partner to whisper a few sentences, one by one, so that you can deduce whether the words involved should be singular or plural. After using the sentences given below, ask your partner to make up others, in the same vein.

BEN AND ELLIE (ARE) GOING HOME
WE BOUGHT (AN) APARTMENT IN SPAIN
WHAT SORT OF CLOTH(ES) DO YOU LIKE?
CHARLOTTE (IS) VERY PRETTY
ALEX GO(ES) TO SCHOOL TOMORROW
THEY (DO) AS THEY LIKE

Exercise 9

Earlier in this chapter, we also looked at conceptual closure, in which life experience can help you to work out what was said. Look at the sentences below and fill in the blanks in several different ways, as long as they make sense. It's important to be open to many possibilities. Some of the options are listed at the end of the exercise. Cover them up while you make your guesses.

1 MY NEW DRESS IS TOO ....
2 THAT GIRL LOOKS REALLY ....
3 IT'S VERY .... IN HERE
4 THOMAS IS THE BEST .... IN THE CLASS
5 DID YOU GO TO THE .... ON YOUR HOLIDAY?
6 HIS FAVOURITE FOOD IS ....

1 tight, slack, bright, short, dirty, small
2 bored, happy, miserable, sad, tired, pretty, young, overweight
3 hot, damp, stuffy, cold, draughty, spacious, dark
4 footballer, looker, sportsman, scholar, writer, chess-player
5 beach, cinema, shops, museum, ski-slopes, carnival
6 chicken, chops, pizza, curry, Chinese, steak, spare ribs

Exercise 10

People with hearing loss often hear things that don't make sense. Try to work out why the sentences below don't make sense, then replace one of the words in each with a word that would look similar on the lips. Cover the correct words at the bottom until you have made all your replacements.

1   THE CHIP WAS AT SEA
2   IT WAS A LOVELY FEW
3   DID YOU PAY THE PILL?
4   I HAVE TOO MUSH TO DO
5   WHAT TIME DID YOU BEAT?
6   I HAVE A HOLE IN MY CHEW
7   HE'S GOING TO LEAF NOW
8   BIKE IS COMING LATER
9   DID YOU SEE THE NEW LAPS?
10   SHE BOUGHT A NEW VEIL CARD

1 ship 2 view 3 bill 4 much 5 meet 6 shoe 7 leave 8 Mike 9 lambs
10 rail

Exercise 11

As mentioned earlier, once you know the topic being discussed, you can help yourself to recognize words by quickly thinking up several words or phrases that might come into play.

Look at the topics listed and try to come up with as many possibilities as you can, concealing the possibilities below until you have finished. Now think of some topics yourself and come up with a list of possibilities.

1 COMPUTERS 2 MOBILE PHONES 3 FOOTBALL 4 FOOD 5 ILLNESS

1   internet, chat rooms, email, software, printer, scanner, keyboard, monitor, search engine, shopping, modem, CD-ROM, hard drive, broadband, games, mouse, USB.
2   texting, messages, voice mail, inbox, phone book, menu, top-up

card, camera phone, multimedia, ring-tone, email, number, speaking, dialling.
3 goal, score, kick, ball, stadium, team, songs, stretcher, cheering, free kick, off-side, tackle, defence, attack, captain, beer, league, foul, champions, injury.
4 breakfast, toast, meal, Chinese, curry, hungry, diet, lunch, cost, café, steak, chips, dinner, hob, recipe, eat, full, salad, restaurant, cookbook, oven, calories, cooker, saucepan, grill.
5 pain, sick, ache, stomach, poorly, hospital, ambulance, doctor, visiting, tablets, bed, tired, paracetamol, hot, flu, sweating, medicine, nurse, consultant, specialist, arthritis, fever, ill, shivering, temperature.

It's fortunate that most conversations stick to each topic for a few minutes at least. However, the subject can change at any time. To help you be aware of the change, you could ask a friend to give you a signal – for example, a discreetly raised finger. If he or she is changing the subject themselves, ask them to introduce it with, 'On another subject …'

Exercise 12

Because it's not possible to lipread every word spoken, it's recommended that you pick out the key words from which you can put the sentence together. Ask a partner to whisper a short sentence and try to read the key words on their lips. The following are examples. Have your partner make up several more.

1 THE DOG WAS CHASING HIS TAIL
2 I'M WORKING A BIT OF OVERTIME TONIGHT
3 WE NEED TO DECORATE THE LOUNGE
4 THE MILK TASTED REALLY SOUR
5 I'VE PUT THAT OLD BLACK COAT IN A CHARITY BAG
6 DO YOU FANCY CHICKEN FOR DINNER?

Key words
1 dog, chasing, tail   2 working, overtime, tonight   3 need, decorate, lounge   4 milk, sour   5 old, coat, charity bag   6 chicken, dinner

Exercise 13

Once you are used to selecting the key words, you need to practise putting them together in a way that makes sense. For each set of words, create at least one sentence that would work, based on the context. Some possibilities are given at the end of the exercise.

1 JAMES	KESTREL	CLIFFS	
2 BABY	NAPPY	CHANGING	
3 LOVE	CD	JAMILIA	
4 STORY	EVACUEES	MAGAZINE	
5 WOMAN	HEEL	CRACK	TILE
6 PHOTO	TAKEN	CHILDREN	AFTERNOON

Possible sentences

1 James saw a kestrel by the cliffs *or* James let the kestrel go by the cliffs.
2 The baby needs her nappy changing *or* Is there a baby nappy changing room?
3 I love that new CD by Jamilia *or* He loves to play that CD by Jamilia.
4 My story about evacuees appeared in a magazine *or* There's a story about evacuees in that magazine.
5 The woman caught her heel in a crack in the tile *or* The woman's heel cracked the tile.
6 I'm having a photo taken of my children this afternoon *or* Her photo was taken with some children this afternoon.

Exercise 14

In this exercise, give a second sentence related to the topic mentioned in the first sentence, as shown in examples 1 and 2 below. Practising with further sentences will help you to forecast what might be said next. However, don't rely solely on guesswork. You must remember to watch the speaker's lips and look for other visual clues.

1 I HATE ALL THOSE TV REALITY SHOWS.
   Example: It's just a cheap way for the TV companies to make money.

2 A CAR RAN INTO THE BACK OF US AT THE LIGHTS.
   Example: We both had whiplash injuries.
3 DID YOU HEAR ABOUT THAT STABBING IN TOWN?
4 IT'S REALLY COLD IN HERE.
5 I HAD THE CAR SERVICED TODAY.
6 THE GARDEN NEEDS WEEDING AGAIN.
7 IS THERE ANYTHING GOOD ON TV TONIGHT?
8 I'D LIKE TO BUY A NEW THREE-PIECE SUITE.

Exercise 15

In this exercise, ask a partner to first read aloud one of the sentences below then whisper a related sentence, while you try to understand it. This will test your skills of association. When you've used the following sentences, ask your partner to make up new ones, speaking the first sentence and only whispering the second, while you try to work it out.

1 MATTHEW FELL ON HIS WAY TO THE SHOPS.
   HE ONLY GRAZED HIS KNEE.
2 WE NEED A NEW FENCE AT THE BOTTOM OF THE GARDEN.
   THE OLD ONE IS FALLING DOWN.
3 DON'T FORGET TO BUY A NEW COLOUR PRINT CARTRIDGE.
   I WANT TO PRINT THOSE PHOTOS I TOOK.
4 WE'RE HAVING SAUSAGE AND BACON.
   WOULD YOU LIKE THEM GRILLED OR FRIED?
5 MY MOTHER WASN'T FEELING VERY WELL.
   I THINK SHE'S CAUGHT THAT VIRUS.
6 I SAW HAZEL REHEARSING FOR THE PLAY.
   SHE'S A VERY GOOD ACTRESS.

Exercise 16

Ensuring that your hearing aid is turned on, look at the following pairs of words that sound very similar to each other. Ask a partner to sit beside you so you are not able to see his or her face. Now your partner should say one of the words, at which you should try to understand it. If you practise this exercise a lot, it will help you to get the most from your hearing aid.

FEND	VEND	DITCH	DISH
MUCH	BUTCH	PAT	BAT
SAVE	SAFE	RAKE	WAKE
LEACH	LEASH	BEEN	MEAN
WOUND	ROUND	THOUGHT	FOUGHT
CHEW	SHOE	SHORE	FOUR
THIRST	FIRST	CODE	ROAD
THUMB	SUM	SIP	ZIP

If you find you're having a problem catching either the beginnings or endings of words, look at whether the difficulty is with specific words. For example, *sip* and *zip* are incredibly similar in sound and on the lips, as are *fend* and *vend*. Indeed, you may always have problems understanding particular words – especially if you can't clearly see the speaker, or if they mumble or have an unfamiliar accent. This is why, rather than relying on lipreading and a hearing aid, speechreading involves looking at the context of the sentence, as well as the speaker's facial expression and other visual cues.

Hearing therapy

This section contains the type of exercises carried out in hearing therapy, which you can either do in conjunction with therapy or alone – depending on how well you believe you are doing and whether you feel you have stalled. Long-term practice with these exercises may work wonders for some people, but others may struggle, not entirely understanding the instructions and concepts. In this case, a referral to a hearing therapist – audiologist or speech–language pathologist – should be requested.

It's also important to extend the exercises, as it's impossible to maintain an improvement by using the same exercise repeatedly. Some may have no problem adding to the exercises given here, but others are less creative and hit a brick wall. A hearing therapist will have an extensive supply of exercise material. However, whether or not you need the additional help of a hearing therapist is entirely your decision. If you're in doubt, seek help. Also, if you don't have a close friend or partner with whom to practise the exercises, it's strongly advised that you have hearing therapy.

Certain listening skills are impossible to practise at home – communication in background noise, for example. A therapist will have equipment that can help you practise these skills. It's also possible to get something wrong and not realize it. A bad habit will be identified very quickly by a therapist. It will then be corrected before it becomes too entrenched in your mind.

To help you deal with difficult emotions regarding your hearing loss, some therapists also offer counselling. It's thought that in most cases group therapy is more effective than one-to-one counselling as you meet other people who share your problem and you can learn from exchanging experiences.

A typical session

A hearing therapy session normally lasts for between one and two hours, and is likely to be held once a week. Although one-to-one sessions sometimes take place, group sessions are more common, involving between four and ten people. The group will probably meet for up to ten weeks.

Some hearing therapy groups deal only with lipreading, which can become boring and is of limited worth. Other groups, however, cover a wider range of techniques, such as conceptual and grammatical closure and visual cues. If you can find a therapist who teaches a variety of techniques, that's the one for you.

The better therapy sessions also offer counselling to help you come to terms with the emotional, social and vocational problems that can occur with hearing loss. Techniques for coping with possible problems are also taught in the better groups. When searching for a good group, always ask for a full breakdown of the therapy they offer.

Learning from others in the same situation as yourself is very important, therefore it's advisable to try to make friends within the group. If you find it difficult to hear the therapist, don't be afraid to say so. Steps will then be taken to ensure you've not missed anything.

If you have very little hearing, even with hearing aids, you would gain more from individual therapy. If you don't have a hearing aid, it's recommended that you postpone therapy until you get one. However, there may be a good reason why you don't own a hearing aid, in which case you should not bypass therapy. It can still be useful.

6

Hearing aids and other audiology equipment

A few weeks after the level of your hearing loss in each ear has been measured and the results plotted on an audiogram, you should be provided with an appropriate hearing aid. A hearing aid amplifies sound, is battery operated, fits in or around your ear and comes in different sizes, shapes and types. It may be very tempting to think of a hearing aid as the first step in solving your communication problems. However, this is not the case. It's important, first of all, to reach emotional acceptance of your hearing problem and to be willing to learn various strategies for coping.

That said, there's no doubt that using a hearing aid is the single most important thing you can do to improve your hearing and that the majority of people who wear one benefit greatly. Unfortunately, as far as the wearer is concerned, there is still a stigma attached to using one – indeed, it's estimated that only 20 per cent of the hearing impaired use one on a regular basis. This is because a hearing aid is usually conspicuous – some people believe it makes them look old and disabled. The embarrassment it causes may even outweigh the benefits. Changing your hairstyle can be enough to hide the aid and restore your confidence – but obviously this is far easier for a woman than a man.

However, due mainly to media attention, few onlookers now believe that a person wearing a hearing aid is not bright – therefore hearing aids are actually losing their stigma. For example, in recent years there have been deaf actresses on *Coronation Street* and the *West Wing*; sign language and lipreading can be seen in the bottom corner of many everyday programmes; hearing impairment has been dealt with on medical programmes, and it has been mentioned many times on TV and radio news programmes, as well as in the newspapers. Another reason why hearing aids are losing their stigma is that 'baby boomers' – people born during the decade after World War II ended and who were teenagers when loud music first became popular – have now reached, or will soon be reaching, hearing-loss age.

A hearing aid cannot give you perfect hearing, but it will make soft sounds louder, enabling speech to be heard and understood more easily and allowing you to hear in situations that caused problems beforehand, such as in a church, bank, loud hall and so on. It should give you the confidence to use the telephone and join in conversations. You may not hear the whole of a conversation, but the sounds you do hear will serve as cues to enable you to fill in the gaps. A hearing aid should also help you to hear high-pitched sounds, such as a child laughing, a bird singing, dishes clashing together in the kitchen, a dog yapping in the distance – which provides the feeling of being in touch with the world around you. You might not like the visibility of a hearing aid, but it does alert others to the fact that you have hearing problems, and should encourage them to make allowances when you misunderstand. It should also encourage others to make an extra effort when speaking to you.

For some people, the controls on the amplifier and microphone are too tiny – very difficult to manage if you suffer from any type of arthritis or have large hands. Many complain that hearing aids are too complicated and that there is often little help available on how best to use them. There's no doubt that it takes time to get used to a hearing aid. To help you become accustomed to the new sounds and the feeling of wearing the aid in your ear, you should gradually build up the amount of time you use it each day. The eventual aim is for you to wear the aid comfortably for most of the day, which may take two or three months to achieve.

Using a hearing aid a lot will not make your hearing deteriorate further, as some might believe. Indeed, if you suffer from tinnitus (see Chapter 7), using a hearing aid can make the noises in your head far less discernible.

Much of the data and guidance in this chapter appears with the permission of the Royal National Institute for Deaf People (RNID). This information is displayed on their invaluable website (the website address and contact details are listed under Useful Addresses at the back of this book).

How do I get a hearing aid?

If you think you have a hearing problem and need a hearing aid, you should see your GP first of all – even if you are considering buying a hearing aid privately and not accepting one free of charge from the National Health Service (NHS). Your GP will ask about your medical history and examine your ears. If there is indeed a problem, you will be referred to either the audiology department at your local hospital or a consultant at the ear, nose and throat (ENT) department. People over 60 may be referred directly to the audiology department without being seen by the ENT department.

Your hearing will then be tested using an audiometer, which produces sounds of different frequencies and levels of loudness. You will tell the audiologist which sounds you can hear and the results are plotted on a chart called an audiogram. It's the audiogram that tells the audiologist whether a hearing aid will help you and, if so, how it should be programmed. The audiologist will need to take an impression of your ear(s) before making an earmould.

Although the NHS has a range of hearing aids, the one for you is likely to depend on your particular hearing loss. Some people may find they can make their selection from two or three kinds. If you are offered two hearing aids – one for each ear – it's recommended that you try them. People with hearing loss often find that two aids work far better than one.

The waiting list for your first NHS hearing aid appointment can vary from between a few weeks to several months. It will be a few weeks after that before the earmould is ready and you are fitted with the aid. At this appointment, the aid will be set to suit your particular hearing requirements and the audiologist will show you how to use and care for it. If you are offered a digital hearing aid, you may be given an appointment to have it fine-tuned within three months, once you are aware of its advantages and disadvantages in different situations.

If you break the aid or have problems using it, contact the audiology department to make an appointment for a repair session or for further instruction. A hearing aid will normally last about five years. Most repairs, including new earmoulds, tubing and batteries, are carried out free of charge on the NHS.

Can I buy a hearing aid privately?

Yes, you can buy privately. The advantages of a private transaction are that you are likely to be provided with a hearing aid far quicker and have a wider choice of aids than from the NHS. In-the-ear aids, for example, are not available on the NHS. You should ask for a recommendation from your GP or a hard-of-hearing friend.

All private dispensers of hearing aids must be registered with the Hearing Aid Council (HAC), the government body responsible for setting standards of professional training, performance and conduct for individuals and companies involved in the assessment of hearing loss and sale of hearing aids. It is a criminal offence for someone who is not registered with the HAC to enter oral negotiations with a view to selling hearing aids. Contact the council for a list of reputable private dispensers in your area (see under Useful Addresses for details of the HAC). It is within your rights to ask for a copy of the HAC's Code of Practice. Qualified dispensers have the letters RHAD after their name, which stands for Registered Hearing Aid Dispenser.

You could also contact the RNID's information line (again, see Useful Addresses) for details of private hearing aid dispensers. However, the RNID cannot recommend one dispenser over another.

Although hearing aids may be cheaper abroad, the RNID would advise you to think carefully before buying overseas as they are unable to recommend any particular models, manufacturers or services. Moreover, seeing the dispenser for adjustments afterwards can be inconvenient and expensive.

Obtaining a hearing aid privately is similar to getting one on the NHS. The hearing aid dispenser you have chosen will test your hearing, provide the aid and show you how to use and care for it. However, you will need to sign a contract agreeing to purchase your chosen hearing aid. As with all legally binding documents, make sure you read the terms and conditions carefully, and check that there's a money-back guarantee. There should be a trial period of at least 28 days, during which you can try out the aid and, if you are not satisfied, return it for a full refund. If the company isn't willing to offer this or offers a guarantee for repairs only, go somewhere else. Check the small print before signing any documents as some companies charge a cancellation fee in excess of 12 per cent.

In choosing your dispenser, it may be wise to compare services and prices. Keep in mind that some dispensers only sell aids from one or two companies, thus limiting your choices, while others sell aids from a wider variety of manufacturers. When making your initial enquiries, ask which companies they represent, and get your quotations in writing, ensuring that they include the cost of hearing tests, the dispenser's time, follow-up appointments and, for behind-the-ear models, the earmould and tubing. You should also ascertain whether there is a discount for buying two aids, if that's what you need.

Home visits from dispensers are not recommended, unless you have no other option. If you do need a home visit, make sure you have someone with you so you don't mishear or feel pressured into buying. It is also important to check that you can easily and quickly contact your chosen dispenser for adjustments and repairs. Using a local dispenser is probably your best option.

The cost

A hearing aid purchased privately will cost between £595 and £3,500 at today's prices, depending on the type and how sophisticated it is. If you have medical insurance, part of the cost may be covered. The discreet in-the-ear and in-the-ear-canal models are generally the most expensive, but may not last as long as other types. You may also have to pay for the initial private hearing test, which is about £25, plus repair costs and for new batteries once the guarantee has run out. Moreover, as a hearing aid lasts only about five years, you will need to buy new ones in the future.

Privately bought hearing aids should be insured against theft, damage and loss.

The analogue hearing aid

Experts in audiology recently commented that the majority of British people with hearing loss are using old-fashioned analogue hearing aids that are 'unusable and poor quality', based on technology that is over 20 years old. Whether a device can be categorized as analogue or digital depends on the technology it uses to process sound waves.

Analogue hearing aids have a built-in microphone that picks up sound and converts it into electrical signals. These signals are amplified and fed to the earphone on the hearing aid, where they are converted back into sounds for you to hear. Unfortunately, as background noise is amplified too, it can be difficult to follow conversations in noisy places. The better analogue devices use automatic gain control (AGC) to magnify quiet sounds (see page 75), but give less amplification to sounds that are already loud. This protects your ears against uncomfortably loud sound levels. However, analogue hearing aids have few of the features that come with advanced digital aids, and you are unlikely to be able to set it very precisely to suit your particular hearing loss.

Body-worn aids and some bone-conduction aids are analogue. Analogue aids are gradually being phased out.

The digital hearing aid

Digital hearing aids look just like analogue aids, but are different in that they process sound by means of a tiny computer chip created to the individual's needs. The hearing aid takes the signal from the microphone and converts it into pieces of data that can be manipulated by the tiny computer, processing sounds very precisely. Digital aids are designed to reduce steady background noise, such as the hum of traffic, the whirr of a fan or the drone of a lawnmower. Listening is therefore less stressful, despite the fact that the aid does not necessarily help you to pick out a single voice from everything else going on.

The more technologically advanced digital aids can be finely adjusted to suit your particular requirements, enabling you to adjust the settings to suit different listening conditions. Some digital aids even make the adjustments automatically. However, not even the best technology available can restore perfect hearing, unlike prescription spectacles that can restore perfect sight. If a digital hearing aid is fitted badly, it is no better than a badly fitted analogue hearing aid.

The company that developed the first digital hearing aid has now brought out the DigiFocus II aid, which makes understanding speech, even in crowded places, far easier than before. The digital process splits all incoming sound, and each frequency is selectively amplified, helping you to separate what you want to hear from distracting background noise. In addition, it amplifies quiet sounds and ensures that loud sounds are not too loud. The DigiFocus II is comfortable and easy to use, with no need to make any adjustments (see Useful Addresses for details).

Some digital hearing aids are designed to reduce whistling – a feature known as 'acoustic feedback suppression' – and others have 'feedback cancellation', which cuts out the whistling that bothers so many hearing aid wearers. These features make the aid easier to use.

Research has shown that, in noisy environments, two factors improve hearing more than anything else. These are: using hearing aids in both ears; and using hearing aids with directional microphones. Both analogue and digital aids come in behind-the-ear, in-the-ear and in-the-ear-canal styles (see page 76). The smaller aids tend to be more awkward and fiddly to use, can break down more easily, and may not feature the loop system (see the section on the 'T' setting, page 74). However, some people find them easier to put in and remove, and of course they're less conspicuous than the larger types.

Directional microphones

The majority of digital hearing aids have microphones that can be set to pick up sounds from in front of you rather than from the side or behind – there is a switch that allows you to hear directional sounds rather than all-round sounds. Hearing only the sounds from in front of you allows you to focus more easily on what you want to listen to in a bustling environment. There are even digital aids that sense automatically where the noise is coming from and adjust the microphone accordingly. Of course, it's impossible for a hearing aid to know what exactly you want to listen to, meaning the lowering of unwanted sound can never be perfect.

Wide dynamic range compression

When a digital hearing aid has a feature called wide dynamic range compression, it can be adjusted independently in each of several bands or channels. It can therefore be programmed to suit your particular hearing deficits and ensures that different sounds are heard at a comfortable volume.

Wide dynamic range compression hearing aids are seldom adjusted automatically. Your audiologist will adjust the settings to suit your requirements when you first receive the hearing aid. If it's not set correctly, you will not get the best out of it. The aid may need fine-tuning by your audiologist once you are used to it.

Availability of digital hearing aids from the NHS

Thanks largely to an RNID campaign to modernize audiology equipment and services, moderate and high-power digital hearing aids with features such as directional microphones, automatic noise reduction and programmes for different listening conditions are now available for adults and children.

Other hearing aid features

Most modern analogue and digital hearing aids have the following features:

The 'T' (telecoil) setting

Both analogue and digital hearing aids may have a telecoil ('T') setting – the telecoil being a tiny component in the aid that picks up signals from a loop system or hearing aid-compatible telephone. Its aim is to make the sound much clearer and cut out background noise. When you receive your hearing aid, ask the audiologist if it has a 'T' setting. Very small aids may not have sufficient room for one, so you won't be able to use it with listening equipment. For example, in-the-ear-canal aids (see page 76) don't have this option.

If your aid has a 'T' setting and you wish to try it out, your audiologist will need to programme it and show you how to switch to it. The 'T' setting can be used with a range of equipment that helps you to hear talks, conversations, plays, shows, the telephone, the TV, the stereo system and so on. There are also conversation aids, radio microphone systems and listening equipment to use with your hearing aid on the 'T' setting.

Automatic gain control

Unfortunately, some older hearing aids amplify all sounds indiscriminately, meaning the louder sounds are uncomfortable to hear. Turning down the volume means that you are also unable to hear quiet sounds. Instead of continually adjusting the volume, it's worth asking your audiologist if you can have a self-adjusting aid.

Most modern analogue and digital aids have a feature called automatic gain control (AGC) that amplifies soft sounds more than loud ones. As a result, soft sounds are audible without the loud sounds being uncomfortably loud. Hearing aids with this feature are sometimes called compression hearing aids because they compress the wide range of sounds they pick up into a smaller range of sounds, which they amplify. Your audiologist should be able to adjust the compression to suit you. If you still find loud sounds too loud, take the aid back to your audiologist for further adjustment. Too much compression means all sounds are of equal volume, preventing you from distinguishing between near and distant sounds, such as someone walking behind you in the street or the different orchestral tones in music. If your hearing aid provides no shades of distance, it needs readjusting.

Multi-band compression

Many modern hearing aids split sound into several frequency bands and apply compression independently in each band – a process called multi-band compression. This allows you to obtain the maximum from your own range of hearing.

Batteries

A quick word about batteries for your hearing aid, which will need regularly replacing. If you own an NHS aid, you can obtain free ones from your local audiology or ENT department with a battery service. They may also be available from your local health centre, and you can buy them from pharmacies.

Behind the ear (BTE) hearing aids

There are several types of hearing aid available. The most common type is the digital behind the ear (BTE) hearing aid, which consists of a piece of moulded plastic – the earmould – that fits the size and shape of your own ear, with the mechanics and battery in a small curved box that sits behind the ear. The two components are connected by a plastic tube.

Instead of having an earmould, there is now the BTE hearing aid called an open ear fitting, with a smaller, soft earpiece at the tip of the tubing. This type of aid is less conspicuous than the ones with an earmould, but is only suitable for mild hearing loss. The sound quality picked up, though, is very natural.

When you take your hearing aid off at night, get into the habit of wiping the earmould, tubing and box with a dry tissue. Alternatively, you could wash the earmould and tubing – not the box – once a week in warm soapy water, before rinsing and drying on a tissue. You will need to blow down the tubing to remove the water, then let it dry overnight. Don't pull the tubing out of the earmould before washing, just pull it off the hooked elbow. The tubing will be prone to splitting, hardening and so on, and will need changing approximately every six months. Be careful to avoid getting the box wet.

In-the-ear (ITE) and in-the-ear-canal (ITC) hearing aids

This type of hearing aid generally has its working parts in the earmould itself, enabling the whole device to fit into your ear. Unfortunately, in-the-ear aids tend to be more prone to malfunctioning than behind-the-ear aids. ITE aids can often be seen from the side, but the smaller ITC aid fits into the ear canal and can barely be seen at all. People with severe hearing loss are unable to benefit sufficiently from this type of aid. Moreover, some people have very narrow ear canals, into which an ITC aid may not fit.

The smaller, custom-made ITE aids should not be washed, but wiped clean with a dry tissue. If your aid has an earmould attached to a hearing aid (the part with the battery in), the earmould can be detached and washed in warm soapy water. Don't get the hearing part wet – just clean it with a dry tissue.

Body-worn hearing aids

There is another, more concealed type of hearing aid – the body-worn aid – where the box containing the microphone and working parts can be attached to your lapel or carried in your pocket, and is connected to the earmould by a wire lead. Body worn hearing aids can be very effective for mild hearing loss, and are useful for people who have problems using tiny switches or buttons.

There is also the type of hearing aid that can be attached to the frame of your spectacles. However, as the aid cannot be taken off, problems arise when the spectacles need repairing or you need a new prescription.

To clean the body-worn aid, wipe it with a dry cloth every time you take it off. The earmould should be washed at least once a week, but the hearing aid should be kept dry.

Bone-conduction hearing aids

Bone-conduction hearing aids are another option, and are mainly used by people who cannot wear a conventional hearing aid due to repeated infections or eczema; because part of their ear or ear canal is missing; or because their ear canal is unusually small. They may also be the best choice for people who suffer from conductive hearing loss (when sound vibrations are unable to pass freely through the outer and middle parts of the ear due to blockage or abnormality of the outer or middle ear).

Unlike conventional hearing aids that send sound into your ear canal, bone conduction hearing aids send sound vibrations through the bones of the skull directly to the inner ear. The individual must wear a headband that holds a tiny bone vibrator in place behind the ear. Obviously, a headband is very visible and puts a lot of people off using this type of device. Also, as the headband needs to be a snug fit to hold the vibrating part tightly to your head, it can be very uncomfortable, causing headaches and soreness. If you wear spectacles, you may prefer to have them strengthened and a bone-conduction aid fitted to them.

Hearing through bone conduction is not as efficient as hearing with the help of a conventional aid (that utilizes sound vibrations and is called an 'air conduction' aid). However, they are far better than no aid at all. Moreover, bone conduction aids generally cut down the number of ear infections you might get, and there is less feedback than from conventional aids.

Bone-anchored hearing aids

The bone-anchored hearing aid (BAHA) also uses bone conduction to improve hearing in people with conductive hearing loss, and removes the need to wear a headband. It provides a better quality of hearing than traditional bone conduction aids and is lighter, more comfortable, less visible, uses fewer batteries and is securely attached. To determine whether a BAHA will work for you, you may be asked to bite on a test rod attached to a BAHA sound processor. Sound is conducted more efficiently through bone than through teeth, so if you can hear the sound, a BAHA will work for you.

A BAHA requires a minor surgical procedure to implant a permanent titanium fixture in the bone behind the ear you hear best with. A small sound processor clips onto this fixture. If your hearing is much the same in both ears and you drive a lot, it would be sensible to choose your left ear so you can more easily have conversations with your passengers. Alternatively, if you use the telephone a lot and are right-handed, it may be better to have the implant fitted behind your right ear.

Four weeks or so after the implant is fitted, you will be shown how to attach and remove the sound processor, how to use the controls and how to clean the area around the fixture. It's important that you, or someone close to you, can keep this area clean to reduce the risk of infection. You won't need further surgery once the fixture has been successfully implanted, but the external parts of the BAHA will need replacing every five years.

This type of aid is suitable for people who are prevented from wearing a conventional aid for the following reasons:

- They have abnormalities of the middle ear or external parts of the ear, or chronic ear infection or inflammation.
- They have hearing loss in both ears for which conventional aids are not suitable.

If you would like to try using a BAHA – which should be free on the NHS – your GP will refer you to the nearest hospital that offers them, but you may have to travel some distance. You will then be assessed to determine whether BAHA will suit you. There are now BAHA support groups where you can meet other people in the same situation as yourself and gain further information and support.

CROS/BiCROS hearing aids

CROS hearing aids are suitable for people who are hard of hearing in only one ear. This type of aid picks up sound from the poor side and feeds it to the better ear. BiCROS hearing aids pick up sound from both sides and feed it to the better ear.

Disposable hearing aids

This type of hearing aid fits right into the ear canal, but as our ear canals are different sizes and shapes and the disposable hearing aid comes in one size only, not everyone is able to use them. The battery lasts for about ten weeks, after which the hearing aid can be disposed of and a new one purchased. Disposable hearing aids can only be bought privately and cost around £26 per month for each ear.

Do I qualify for a digital hearing aid?

If you think you would benefit from using a digital hearing aid, but have never owned a hearing aid before, you need first to see your GP, who will refer you to a local audiology department. You may be offered a digital hearing aid for each ear, in which case it would be wise to give them a good try. The majority of people hear better when using two hearing aids.

People who already have analogue hearing aids and would like to try a digital aid can be reassessed by their audiology department. Go back to your GP first of all, to ask for a referral.

War pensioners who were awarded the pension for deafness resulting from their time in service are always put to the top of the hearing aid waiting list. They are seen more promptly at the audiology clinic but are not entitled to better hearing aids than other patients.

If you have purchased a hearing aid privately in the past, you will still qualify for an NHS hearing aid.

People who do not qualify for a digital hearing aid

The people who are generally not eligible for digital hearing aids are as follows:

- Those who have been fitted with a new hearing aid within the last three years and have no significant deterioration in hearing capacity. If your hearing has deteriorated significantly, however, you should be eligible to receive a new digital aid.
- Those who already own an NHS hearing aid, in which case you should wait to be invited to the clinic for a review of your condition. However, if you are struggling to use the aid, you should ask for an appointment.
- Those who live overseas, who generally don't qualify for an NHS hearing aid.
- Those who live outside an area for which a particular hospital provides a service, in which case you are unlikely to be accepted onto their hearing aid waiting list.

Other important points

If you want to use a digital aid from the NHS, it's important to be aware of the following points:

- After being awarded a digital aid, you will be sent a follow-up appointment.
- Hearing aid batteries and repairs are free of charge.
- NHS hearing aids are always government property so can't be declared on your household insurance.
- If you lose or damage a digital aid, you may be asked to pay some of the cost toward a replacement aid.
- If you no longer need your hearing aid, you should return it to your audiology department.

How to get the best from your hearing aid

To get the best from the aid, follow these important steps:

- When you receive your hearing aid, it's vital that you take time to practise putting it in your ear and using the various controls. The earmould should fit snugly, but be comfortable once you get used to the feel of it. Initially, try wearing it for about an hour a day, at a time when there is little background noise. Get used to everyday noises such as taps running, the kettle boiling and doors opening and shutting. In quiet surroundings, practise conversations with one person.
- When you are used to conversations with one person, try speaking with two, three or four people – again in quiet surroundings. Don't allow yourself to be upset if you aren't able to catch all that is said. It's good enough if, at this point, you can follow the general thread of the conversation. With more practice, you should be able to catch more.
- When you are satisfied with the way your hearing aid helps you indoors, try using it outdoors. Avoid having the volume too high as some outdoor noises can be very loud.
- When you are satisfied that you can benefit from your hearing aid indoors and outdoors, try using it in a pub, restaurant, shopping centre or other noisy place. Don't be discouraged when you struggle to hear all of a conversation – it should become easier in time.
- If you can't get accustomed to using the aid, ask your GP for a referral to your audiologist or private hearing aid dispenser. It

may take a little extra help and advice to set you on the right track.

Cochlear implants

A cochlear implant is a small complex electronic device that is surgically implanted under the skin behind the ear. Such implants are offered only to people who are severely hard of hearing or profoundly deaf. They help to provide a sense of sound, give a person a useful auditory understanding of the environment and assist them in understanding speech. However, cochlear implants cannot restore or create normal hearing.

An implant consists of these four basic parts:

- a microphone, worn as a box behind the ear, to pick up sounds. The microphone is connected by tiny wires to a transmitter inside the ear;
- a speech processor to select and arrange the sounds picked up by the microphone;
- a transmitter and receiver/stimulator to receive signals from the speech processor and convert them into electrical impulses;
- electrodes to collect the electrical impulses and relay them to the brain.

Unlike hearing aids that amplify normal sounds, cochlear implants pick up useful sounds as electrical impulses and transmit them to the brain. Hearing through a cochlear implant sounds different from normal hearing, but once you have learned to interpret the sounds correctly, you should be able to communicate very well, and to use the telephone effectively.

Currently, who gets cochlear implants?

Children and adults whose inner ear hair cells are abnormal or have been irreparably damaged can be offered this type of implant. A deaf child may be offered one to help him or her to acquire speech, language, developmental and social skills, the implant being coupled with intensive post-implantation therapy. Experts are undecided on the best age for implantation, but most children who receive them are between two and six years old. It appears that earlier implantation is more effective. However, some parties disapprove of cochlear implants being fitted in small children on the grounds that it is interfering with nature. As mentioned earlier, it's also a fact that people who are born deaf tend not to isolate themselves or become depressed. They generally socialize with others in the same situation and get a lot out of life. There are always times when they need to deal with hearing people, though, and this may cause problems.

Adults who have lost all their hearing, usually in later life, may also be offered cochlear implants, and are more able than children to associate the sounds they hear through the implant with sounds they remember from their hearing days. As a result, they are more likely to understand speech without visual cues, speechreading or sign language.

According to the Food and Drug Administration, almost 100,000 people worldwide had received cochlear implants by 2005.

How do you get a cochlear implant?

If you think a cochlear implant may be your best option, you need to discuss this with your GP and audiologist. Provided that they are in agreement with you, the final decision will involve discussions with other medical professionals, including a surgeon. The implant and surgical procedure is very expensive and medical professionals need to feel assured that you will benefit from it. The procedure is as safe as any surgery can be, but complications do occur in some people, and you need to be aware of this. You should also be prepared for the time and patience required as you learn to interpret the sounds created by the implant. Speech–language pathologists and audiologists will help you with this. It's also important to know that not everyone can effectively interpret the sounds. Most interpret them very well, but a small number of people have difficulties.

A new development

I'm pleased to say that advancements in cochlear implant technology are occurring all the time. For example, a cochlear implant that should enable deaf people to hear music is an exciting prospect, given that existing implants allow people to listen far more easily to speech than music. Commercial use of this implant is at least ten years away, but it should give users manual control over the frequencies they hear, allowing them also to tune in to individuals in noisy surroundings. According to *New Scientist* magazine (October 2005), there would be no need to wear a box behind the ear as the whole implant could be put into the ear. Its design is not dissimilar to a comb, with a row of bar-shaped elements that resonate like a tuning fork in response to sound. The piezoelectric coating of the bars (piezoelectric means a small crystal device that creates an electric current) gives rise to an electrically generated pulse that is relayed directly to the auditory nerve in the cochlea.

The prototype of this implant measures two square centimetres, which is still fairly large. The challenge now for researchers is to miniaturize the elements so that the implant can fit into the cochlea and still resonate at audible frequencies.

7

Tinnitus

Tinnitus is a common physical problem, and can arise at any age. The condition is characterized by the sensation of noises heard in your head, when no such external physical noise is present. The noises vary in different people, some hearing more than one sound. Such noises include ringing, buzzing, hissing, whistling, roaring, humming and machine-type noises – in fact, tinnitus comes from the Latin word *tinnire*, which means to imitate a ring or tinkle. The noises are also variable, changing in loudness and character on occasion.

Continually to hear noises in your head can be very distressing, and as the noises are more noticeable in a very quiet environment, getting a good night's sleep is a problem for many. Prolonged tinnitus can even cause the individual to panic and fear a severe, chronic illness.

People with moderate to severe tinnitus combined with hearing loss can blame their tinnitus for their hearing problems, particularly when communicating in groups or when there is background noise. However, tinnitus is often a symptom of hearing loss. It is certainly not the cause.

The condition can also, in extreme cases, be very debilitating, affecting the person's ability to work and cope with a normal active life. People with tinnitus may also suffer from the following:

- extreme distress and even thoughts of suicide;
- frequent mood swings;
- anxiety and depression;
- tension, irritability and frustration;
- poor concentration;
- difficulty sleeping.

In some people, the condition is constant, fluctuating with stress or tiredness. In others it comes and goes. After spending time at a loud nightclub or concert, many people experience buzzing in their ears – however, this type of tinnitus is generally temporary, disappearing within 48 hours.

Estimates of prevalence vary, but it's believed that the majority of people experience tinnitus at some stage in their lives. Between 15 and 20 per cent of the population in industrialized countries suffer from problematic tinnitus, 8 per cent of whom feel it greatly impinges on their daily lives. Of that number, 0.5 to 1 per cent report that their symptoms are so pronounced that they are prevented from leading a normal life. As yet, though, there is no way to determine objectively whether a person has noises in the ear and, if so, how loud they are. Instead, doctors must rely on the information given them by the patient.

Two leading charities – the Royal National Institute for Deaf People (RNID) and the British Tinnitus Association (BTA) – recently conducted an internet survey in which 40 per cent of the 900 respondents reported that tinnitus had a negative impact on their professional lives and personal relationships. They added that a lack of understanding from a partner compounded the problem. Furthermore, over 10 per cent said the condition had affected their sex drive.

The RNID and BTA can offer support and advice to people with tinnitus. Sufferers should also visit their GP, who can provide help and advice, as well as a referral to a specialist.

Oversensitivity to sounds (hyperacusis)

It is estimated that 45 per cent of people with tinnitus experience some discomfort when hearing moderately loud sounds, and that a smaller percentage are ultra-sensitive to sounds the ear is normally able to tolerate – a condition known as *hyperacusis*. These everyday sounds may include a dog barking some way down the street, music at a normal volume and a car passing by. For these people, noise from a vacuum cleaner, loud music, carpentry and construction work is extremely painful to the ears. The condition can be accompanied by hearing loss, dizziness, severely disturbed sleep, difficulty in concentrating, anxiety, depression and social withdrawal. Hyperacusis is not limited to individuals who are hard of hearing. Indeed, it is often experienced by people with only a slight loss in hearing – so small that they may not even be aware of it.

The severity of hyperacusis ranges from mild to profound and is usually more severe in one ear than the other. In many cases, however, both ears are eventually affected. The condition can arise after a head injury, when the swelling, congestion, bleeding and bruising have all subsided. Hyperacusis may also be related to an autoimmune disorder (where the immune system attacks the body's own cells) such as in various skin conditions, allergies and arthritis. Individuals with other inflammatory conditions are also believed to be susceptible to developing hyperacusis.

Many people with hyperacusis resort to wearing earplugs, even for normal conversation. Of course, this can then interfere with the amount of speech they are able to hear. It is advisable that sufferers gradually reduce the amount of hearing protection they use – a sudden removal can be very uncomfortable. Special non-linear earplugs may be recommended by your audiologist as they reduce the impact of sudden loud sounds while allowing the quieter sounds to filter through.

Habituation therapy – which entails retraining the part of the brain involved in tinnitus by the prolonged use of low-level broadband noise or amplified environmental sound – can not only reduce the perception of tinnitus, it can also limit hyperacusis. This has even greater benefit when used in conjunction with counselling.

Ask your doctor, audiologist or ENT specialist for more information on these matters. Family and friends of the person can help by reducing loud noises in the home, workplace or social gatherings. It is also important for others to understand why the individual might try to avoid noisy situations.

Three stages of tinnitus

Tinnitus is often linked with hearing loss as it is usually the result of damage to one or more of the components of the ear (see page 88). The condition consists of three stages, as shown below:

- *Generation* – This usually involves deterioration of the cochlea or the auditory nerve, and can be caused by noise exposure or taking certain prescription medications (see pages 89–90).
- *Detection* – The brain detects the change in nerve activity, which is perceived as sound.
- *Evaluation* – When the emotional and reflex centres of the brain assess the sound and perceive it as threatening, tinnitus becomes a problem.

Causes

Research has shown that deterioration of the cochlea hair cells involved in hearing can play a significant role in the onset of tinnitus. There are also numerous other possible causes, including high blood pressure, damage to the temperomandibular joint (lower jaw joint), diseases of the cervical (upper) spine, heart valve problems, cholesterol problems, anaemia, previous inflammatory conditions such as rubella, toxoplasmosis or flu, underactive thyroid gland, diabetes, blockage in the auditory canal, constriction of blood vessels, prolonged middle ear infections, inflammation of the carotid artery, swelling of the blood vessel in the ear, Meniere's disease (swelling of a duct in the ear) and tumours in the inner ear, auditory nerve, brain stem or auditory cortex of the brain.

However, many long-term sufferers have never experienced any of these things and the root cause remains a mystery. Disruption of the hair cells in the cochlea is the chief problem in the majority of cases, and can arise for a variety of reasons.

It is important to note that tinnitus is rarely linked to a serious disorder and individuals often learn to manage it effectively.

Malfunctioning frequencies

The hair cells within the cochlea are the most important sense organs in the auditory system, for they send sound vibrations to the auditory nerve (see Chapter 1). In turn, the vibrations are relayed to the brain, various areas of which interpret the sounds in different ways. When the hair cells are damaged for some reason, malfunctions in one or more sound frequencies result. The brain attempts to compensate for this by increasing the damaged frequency range, actively inhibiting nerve cells that suppress the functioning of frequencies at the parameters of the damaged range.

This is a difficult concept to grasp and can perhaps be better explained by imagining three loudspeakers in the brain, one of which – the bass, for example – starts to malfunction. In attempting to compensate for this, the brain tries to increase the frequency range of the defective loudspeaker, which it does by dampening down the frequencies at the edges of the damaged range. The sounds a person would hear from the malfunctioning frequencies are halted, but instead the brain's blocking signals that dampen them can actually be heard, and is what we know as tinnitus. The blocking signals are heard only faintly at first, but can grow louder, with time.

Noise exposure

Long-term exposure to loud noise can not only lead to hearing loss, it is also the most commonly known cause of tinnitus. In 2002, the RNID sponsored research into tinnitus and young adults who regularly go clubbing, and it was found that a staggering three-quarters experience temporary tinnitus. Those who continue to expose themselves to loud noise over a prolonged period are at risk of developing permanent tinnitus. If you work in a noisy environment, it's advisable to ensure that your employers follow the 'noise at work' regulations, which include issuing ear protection and giving employees frequent breaks from the noise.

In the tinnitus survey mentioned, more than 20 per cent of respondents blamed noise in the workplace for the onset of their condition.

Medications

Tinnitus is listed as a side effect of some prescribed medications, including streptomycin, gentamicin, diuretics, steroids, heart medicines, anaesthetics, quinine and aspirin-containing drugs. However, not everyone who takes these particular medications develops tinnitus, or finds it getting worse. It may be that the disorder for which you are taking the medication is causing or worsening your tinnitus or, in fact, that the cause could be the stress provoked by the disorder. If you have developed tinnitus after taking a particular medication, it's advisable to see your GP, who may agree to your trying a different medication or reducing the quantity of your current medication.

A small number of prescribed medications are capable of damaging the ear or hearing and are described as *ototoxic*. However, ototoxic medications are generally only prescribed to treat a life-threatening illness. In such cases, the risk of side effects is outweighed by the necessity to save the person's life. When ototoxic medications are prescribed, the patient should be carefully monitored. Such medicines include heart and chemotherapy drugs.

Stress

Stress cannot directly cause tinnitus, but it can raise its volume. Tinnitus is thus often a warning sign of physical strain or emotional stress and trauma. We all have some stress in our lives. It's when we experience significant periods of stress or stressful events occur, such as the death of a loved one or injury in an accident, that tinnitus can become a problem. Hearing noises in your ear can, in itself, be stressful. For that reason it's important to learn to manage the stress.

Factors that can worsen tinnitus

In addition to stress and noise exposure, other common exacer-bating factors include drinking a lot of alcohol, the nicotine from cigarette and cigar smoking and drinking large amounts of caffeine.

A cross-sectional study found that current smokers were 1.69 times more likely to have hearing loss than non-smokers (Cruickshanks, 1998). Non-smoking participants who lived with a smoker were more likely to have hearing loss than those who were not exposed to cigarette or cigar smoke in the home.

Managing tinnitus

If it's not possible to identify and therefore treat the condition underlying tinnitus, there are ways to manage the problem success-fully. For instance, habituation therapy helps individuals to adapt gradually to their tinnitus so that, ultimately, attention is not (or seldom) given to sounds that were previously so disturbing. In time, emotional acceptance is achieved. Other management techniques are hearing aids, sound therapy, relaxation and counselling.

Distraction

During the day, listening to TV, the radio or music generally allows tinnitus sounds to move into the background. It's seldom either possible or acceptable to listen to such sounds all day, in which case reading a book or concentrating on your work can be effective distractions. However, if you find you can't read or work because of the noises in your head, having soft music in the background or using a sound generator (see below) should help. An inexpensive option is to use FM radio static – the hissing sound that comes when the radio is tuned between stations. This sound is known as white noise.

Sound therapy (masking)

The awareness of tinnitus is greater in quiet surroundings, such as in bed at night. However, in a constant low background noise the sounds seem to diminish greatly. In effect, our senses are not reacting to the real value of the sounds, but rather to the difference between the sounds and the background. Scientists have therefore found that the most important approach to tinnitus management is the presence of a neutral sound that is easily ignored.

Sound therapy involves listening to a sound you find pleasant, such as background radio or TV and tranquil sounds from a relaxation CD – in the form of soft music, gentle rainfall or waves lapping against a pebble beach. With severe tinnitus, a sound generator can supply a gentle hissing sound, or low-level white noise that provides a constant bland, neutral sound that is easily ignored and which effectively masks the tinnitus sounds. Sound generators look like hearing aids and fit either behind or inside the ear. Such devices can run on batteries as well as mains electricity. However, you will need to be fitted for one by your audiologist or ENT specialist.

Masking tinnitus is not considered a form of treatment for the condition, but it can provide relief in the short term – perhaps sufficient to allow you to fall asleep at night. During the periods of light sleep we all have every night, the use of a sound generator makes it less likely that the tinnitus will wake you. When trying to fall asleep, avoid focusing on the low-level sound. Instead, allow it to fade into the background of your awareness.

Hearing aids

People who have hearing loss combined with tinnitus will usually find benefit for both conditions by using a hearing aid. Because they amplify the sounds around you, hearing aids can mask tinnitus sounds, help to compensate for your hearing loss and stop you from straining to hear conversations. If you can adapt to the amplification provided by the hearing aid, the reduction in the stress and fatigue resulting from the tinnitus sounds and not being able to hear conversations is a great bonus in all areas of your life.

In quieter surroundings, hearing aids may be less effective as a tinnitus management tool. You may also need to use a sound generator or distraction technique.

Counselling

If you have tried the above tinnitus management techniques and still feel distressed by the noises in your head, it's important that you seek counselling – or cognitive behavioural therapy (also known as CBT) – for the problem. Counselling can help you to learn to live with tinnitus – known as *habituation*. Habituation is defined as the reduction of an innate response to a frequently repeated stimulus. It works by changing your sound response systems so that you eventually become less aware of the noise.

Discussing your tinnitus and explaining how it affects your life can also be of benefit. Counselling can also help with the following:

- understanding how tinnitus arises;
- understanding that the condition does not put you at risk in any way;
- learning ways of focusing your attention away from your tinnitus;

- changing your reactions to the noises and so allowing you to control the stress associated with tinnitus.

Relaxation and hypnotherapy

Because tinnitus can be very frustrating and distressing, a useful form of self-help is to follow a daily relaxation routine. This can enable you to tone down your instinctive responses when you start to become anxious.

Many people with tinnitus find that hypnotherapy can help indirectly by encouraging relaxation (there's more information about relaxation and hypnotherapy in Chapter 8).

8

Complementary therapies

Many people with hearing loss use complementary therapies. However, some can cause adverse reactions and their quality and strength is not controlled by a regulating body. In comparison with mainstream medicine, where there has been a vast amount of research, there has been very little research and few controlled scientific trials into the effects of complementary medicine. Before deciding to try a particular therapy, it is recommended that you find out as much as you can about it. You could also ask your doctor's advice.

That said, some people with hearing loss who use complementary therapies report great benefits. However, the benefits may, to some extent, come from individuals knowing they are doing something positive to help themselves. There is no doubt that complementary therapies can reduce the anxiety, anger, frustration, stress, depression and so on that come with impaired hearing; and the absence of these negative emotions can make it appear easier to hear.

Some of the most commonly used forms of therapy – excluding prayer – are natural, such as deep-breathing exercises and meditation. Visits to complementary medicine practitioners vastly outnumber the total number of visits to doctors and other medical professionals, according to a 1997 survey. The most common reason for using complementary therapy was that the patient believed it would be helpful when combined with conventional treatments.

Deafness Research UK, together with major research fundraisers such as the Medical Research Council, are welcoming research proposals into the effects of complementary medicine on hearing loss. Where there is a psychological component to hearing loss – as there invariably is – Deafness Research UK believes that the more relaxing therapies can be of great benefit.

Tinnitus often responds well to complementary therapies – particularly hypnotherapy, relaxation and meditation.

Acupuncture

An ancient form of oriental healing, acupuncture involves puncturing the skin with fine needles at specific points in the body. These points are located along energy channels (meridians) that are believed to correspond with certain internal organs. This energy is known as chi. Needles are inserted to increase, decrease or unblock the flow of chi energy so that the balance of yin and yang is restored.

Yin, the female force, is calm and passive; it also represents dark, cold, swelling and moisture. On the other hand, yang, the male force, is stimulating and aggressive, representing heat, light, contraction and dryness. It is thought that an imbalance in these forces is the cause of illness and disease. For example, a person who feels the cold, suffers fluid retention and fatigue would be considered to have an excess of yin. A person suffering from repeated headaches, however, will be deemed to have an excess of yang. Emotional, physical or environmental factors are believed to disturb the chi energy balance, and can also be treated.

A qualified acupuncturist will use a set method to determine acupuncture points – it is thought there are as many as 2,000 acupuncture points on the body. At a consultation, questions may be asked about lifestyle, sleeping patterns, fears, phobias, and reactions to stress. The pulses will be felt, then the acupuncture itself carried out, fine needles being placed in the relevant sites. The first consultation will normally last for an hour, and the client should notice a change for the better after four to six sessions.

There are many anecdotal reports of improvements in hearing as a result of acupuncture treatments. Indeed, acupuncturists inform us that treatment of clients with sensorineural hearing loss can boost the circulation of fluids in the head and so improve hearing. However, in a study of 29 volunteers with stable bilateral (both ears affected) sensorineural hearing loss, each subject received 30 acupuncture treatments (Abel, 1976). During the year following treatment, significant improvements in hearing were not found. It seems the study was looking for *significant* improvements, which suggests that any small improvements were not noted. Clearly, there is a need for further investigation. Acupuncture can certainly reduce the stress and anxiety linked to hearing loss, and that can allow some to catch more of the spoken word.

Acupuncture is a safe therapy. The only very slight risk is that of infection from the needles.

Aromatherapy

Certain health disorders can be treated by stimulating our sense of smell with aromatic oils – known as essential oils. Once stimulated, it is believed that a particular smell can help to treat a particular health problem. There's no doubt at all that aromatherapy can aid relaxation and help to reduce anxiety, tension and depression, which often accompany hearing loss.

Concentrated essential oils are extracted from plants and may either be inhaled, rubbed directly into the skin or used in bathing. Each odour relates to its plant of origin – lavender oil has the aroma of the lavender plant, geranium the aroma of the geranium plant, and so on.

Plant essences have been used for healing throughout the ages, smaller amounts being used for aromatherapy purposes than for herbal medicines. The highly concentrated aromatherapy oils are obtained either by steaming a particular plant extract until the oil glands burst, or by soaking the plant extract in hot oil so that the cells collapse and release their essence.

Techniques used in aromatherapy

There are several ways of using aromatherapy. The main ones are as follows:

- *Inhalation* – Giving the fastest result, inhalation of essential oils has a direct influence on the olfactory (nasal) organs, which is immediately received by the brain. Steam inhalation is the most popular technique. This can be achieved either by mixing a few drops of oil with a bowlful of boiling water, or by using an oil burner, whereby a tea-light candle heats a small container of water into which a few drops of oil has been added.

- *Massage* – Essential oils intended for massage are normally pre-diluted. They should never be applied directly to the skin in an undiluted (pure) form. When using undiluted essential oils, mix three or four drops with a neutral carrier oil such as olive or safflower oil. After penetrating the skin, the oils are absorbed by the body, exerting a positive influence on a particular organ or set of tissues.
- *Bathing* – Tension and anxiety can be reduced by using aroma-therapy oils in the bath. A few drops of pure essential oil should be added directly to running tap water – it disperses and mixes more efficiently this way. No more than twenty drops of oil in total should be used.

Ear infections

If you suffer from repeated infections of the outer ear and ear canal, you should ask your GP whether it is safe for you to self-treat with aromatherapy oils. Use of the oils can relieve the inflammation and pain of an infection.

People who suffer from the more serious infections of the middle and inner ear should seek medical treatment. You may still be able to use essential oils, but only under the guidance of your GP. It's important to note that a perforated ear drum should not be self-treated. This can cause more harm than good.

Lavender, tea tree and Roman chamomile oils are undoubtedly the most useful for treating infection and can be made up into ear oil with the following recipe:

- 8 drops lavender oil
- 8 drops tea tree oil
- up to 4 drops Roman chamomile oil (optional)
- 1 tbsp olive oil or sweet almond oil (the carrier oil)

Blend the oils well, then rub a little of the blend around the outside of your ear and also down the side of your neck. When you make a bottle of oil for use on other occasions, remember to label the bottle.

If your ear infection is due to a cold or flu, which is likely to cause congestion in your upper respiratory tract, you may obtain relief from inhaling a mixture of peppermint and eucalyptus – 8 drops of each mixed with a carrier oil.

Hearing loss

It has been reported that using a blend of the oils in the following recipes has improved hearing loss to some degree. These reports are purely anecdotal, however.

Recipe 1

- 10 drops cypress
- 10 drops helichrysum
- 10 drops marjoram
- 10 drops Roman chamomile
- 1 fluid ounce olive or sweet almond oil (the carrier oil)

Recipe 2

- 15 drops marjoram
- 10 drops helichrysum
- 10 drops Roman chamomile
- 3 drops rosemary
- 1 fluid ounce olive oil or sweet almond oil (the carrier oil)

For each individual recipe, blend the essential oils listed and add to the carrier oil. Apply a few drops of the blend to the ear, the ear canal and down on to the neck area around the ear. Use 2–4 times a day until you notice an improvement. However, avoid using for more than 10 days at a time.

Relaxation

Lavender is the most popular oil for relaxation. It is a wonderful restorative and excellent for relieving tension headaches as well as stress. However, there are several others that when used alone or blended can provide a relaxing atmosphere – Roman chamomile and ylang ylang, for example. Ylang ylang has relaxing properties, a calming effect on the heartbeat rate and can relieve palpitations and raised blood pressure. Chamomile can also be very soothing, and aids both sleep and digestion.

Drop relaxation oils into the vessel part of the burner and top up with water. Light the tea light candle and try to relax while the essential oils scent the whole room – don't let the water evaporate totally. Such oils are safe around babies and children, as rather than being overpowering, the aroma is soft and soothing.

Recipe 1

- 5 drops lavender
- 2 drops Roman chamomile
- 1 drop ylang ylang
- Blend well and diffuse in a burner

Recipe 2

- 8 drops mandarin
- 3 drops neroli
- 3 drops ylang ylang
- Blend well and diffuse in a burner

Recipe 3

- 10 drops bergamot
- 2 drops rose otto
- 3 drops Roman chamomile
- Blend well and diffuse in a burner

Relaxation recipes 2 and 3 can be added to two ounces of distilled water, shaken well and used in a spray bottle for a room freshener with relaxing properties.

Recipe 4

For relaxation, this is a great blend for use in the bath.

- 3 drops lavender
- 2 drops marjoram
- 2 drops basil
- 1 drop vetiver
- 1 drop fennel

Seeing an aromatherapist

Because aromatherapy is a holistic therapy (where the practitioner looks at the person and his or her ills as a whole), questions on lifestyle, family circumstances and so on will be asked by your chosen therapist. Depending upon your answers, a suitable blend of oils will be recommended and a back massage offered. As well as being beneficial health-wise, aromatherapy massages are very relaxing. If you are unable to consult with a qualified aromatherapist, your local health food store may provide you with details of which essential oils are appropriate for your needs. Alternatively, you may want to borrow a good aromatherapy book from your library.

Homeopathy

The homeopathic approach to medicine is holistic – that is, the overall health of a person, physical, emotional and psychological, is assessed before treatment commences. The homeopathic belief is that the whole make-up of a person determines the disorders to which he or she is prone, and the symptoms likely to occur. After a thorough consultation, the homeopath will offer a remedy compatible with the patient's symptoms as well as with his or her temperament and characteristics. Consequently, two individuals with the same disorder may be offered entirely different remedies.

Homeopathic remedies are derived from plant, mineral and animal substances, which are soaked in alcohol to extract the 'live' ingredients. This initial solution is then diluted many times, being vigorously shaken each time to add energy. Impurities are removed and the remaining solution made up into tablets, ointments, powders or suppositories. Low-dilution remedies are used for severe symptoms while high-dilution remedies are used for milder symptoms.

The homeopathic concept has, since antiquity, been that 'like cures like'. The full healing abilities of this type of remedy were first recognized in the early nineteenth century when a German doctor, Samuel Hahnemann, noticed that the herbal cure for malaria – which was based on an extract of cinchona bark (quinine) – actually produced symptoms of malaria. Further tests convinced him that the production of mild symptoms caused the body to fight the disease. He went on to treat malaria patients successfully with dilute doses of cinchona bark.

Each homeopathic remedy is first 'proved' by being taken by a healthy person – usually a volunteer homeopath – and the symptoms noted. This remedy is said to be capable of curing the same symptoms in an ill person. The whole idea of 'proving' and using homeopathic remedies can be difficult to comprehend, as it is exactly the opposite of how conventional medicines operate. For example, a patient who has a cold with a runny nose would be treated with a homeopathic remedy that would produce a runny nose in a healthy patient. Conventional medicine, on the other hand, would provide something that blocks up the nose.

Homeopaths claim that, nowadays, a remedy can be formulated to aid virtually every disorder, including sensorineural hearing loss and tinnitus. Although remedies are safe and non-addictive, occasionally the patient's symptoms may briefly worsen. This is known as a 'healing crisis' and is usually short-lived. It is actually a good indication that the remedy is working well.

It is a common misconception that you can just pop along to your local chemist, look up your particular complaint on the homeopathic remedy chart, and begin taking the remedy. If only it were that simple … Homeopathic training takes several years, and a lot of knowledge and experience is required before practitioners can decide the correct remedies for complaints other than the very superficial. And, as I mentioned earlier, homeopathy is specific to each individual. What works for one person is not liable to work for another.

Hypnotherapy

For several decades it's been known that hypnotherapy is capable of reducing stress, anxiety and phobias. Recent studies have shown that it's also effective in the treatment of depression. When stress and depression are features of hearing impairment, hypnotherapy is an avenue well worth exploring. It can make all the difference to your ability to cope.

In the treatment of tinnitus, it would seem that hypnotherapy is the best therapy option. Hypnotherapists claim that it can eliminate the problem in some people and reduce the associated volume, stress and other negative emotions in others. In fact, in a recent study of hypnotherapy as a treatment for tinnitus, 73 per cent reported that the noises had either disappeared or were greatly reduced.

The reason that more people with tinnitus don't pursue hypnotherapy is its negative media perception. One common fear is that the therapist may, while you are in a trance state, implant dangerous suggestions, or extract improper personal information. I can only stress that patients can come out of the trance at any time – particularly if they are asked to do or say something they would not even contemplate when awake. Malpractice would only have to be brought to light once to ruin the therapist's career.

Hypnotherapy is, as the name states, about the hypnotist using the power of hypnotism for therapeutic purposes. The person under hypnosis is in a state of heightened awareness and focused concentration – scientifically measurable by instruments and known as the alpha state. Scientific research has shown this state of mind to be superior for learning, memory recall and training the mind to overcome negative programming, including a stressful reaction to tinnitus and hearing loss. During hypnotherapy, the therapist attempts to remove the emotional response from certain associations. Once that has been done, he or she can help the unconscious mind to focus on stimuli other than the tinnitus, or the stress a hearing-impaired person experiences in group situations.

For tinnitus in particular, one form of hypnotherapy is regression therapy, where the client is taken back to the time before the onset of tinnitus to discover the trigger of the noise. Hypnotherapists claim that the trigger can be found in most cases, after which the client will be guided into repeatedly experiencing the cause. Eventually the emotional impact will become boring, or even amusing. Another method involving regression is to bring the trigger of tinnitus into the client's awareness so they can make a cognitive decision regarding how they feel about the condition. At this point, the tinnitus will reduce or disappear for many people.

Another form of hypnotherapy is suggestion, which is usually offered in combination with regression therapy, or as an alternative if the trigger can't be found. With suggestion, the hypnotherapist offers unconscious suggestions such as, for a client with tinnitus, 'On returning to your wide awake state of mind, you will notice the noise that was so distracting earlier will now be very faint. This will enable you to lead a more peaceful life and spend more time relaxing ...'

After the first session, the therapist may recommend that you purchase an audio recording to allow you to self-hypnotize on a daily basis. Self-hypnosis has been studied on several occasions and the average improvement rate lies between 60 and 75 per cent.

Through the Yellow Pages and/or the internet you will be able to find the numbers of several hypnotherapists in your area. You should call each one first to ask if they know what tinnitus is. If they do, enquire whether they think they can help you and which type of therapy they would use exactly. The charge is generally reasonable and hypnotherapists tend to be kindly, attentive people.

Indian head massage

The stress, anxiety and tension provoked by hearing loss and tinnitus can be reduced by regular Indian head massage. This involves using controlled caresses known as the comb, root pull and spider walk. The massage is concentrated primarily on the face and scalp, but can also be applied to the upper back, neck, shoulders and upper arms.

Indian head massage originated in India over a thousand years ago and is said to have an intense effect on the chakras that govern the mind, body and spirit – the three most important chakras. We are all said to possess seven chakras, which are energy vortexes we require to continue striving. On being given an Indian head massage, a client experiences a release of tension almost immediately. Indeed, clients are invariably surprised at how quickly and thoroughly they relax. It is claimed that the technique is also beneficial for the following:

- it can relieve tension headaches and migraines;
- it encourages the body to rest and helps to promote sleep;
- it eases dizziness and vertigo;
- it helps to ease mental fatigue and promote clearer thinking and concentration;
- it helps to relieve depression;

- in some cases, it is said to improve sensorineural hearing loss by increasing fluid flow through the brain;
- it promotes a feeling of balance and calm.

Many people who use Indian head massage on a regular basis have described it as 'magical' in its relaxing effects.

Reflexology

Reflexology, an ancient oriental therapy, was not adopted in the western world until fairly recently. It operates on the proposition that the body is divided into different energy zones, all of which can be exploited in the prevention and treatment of any disorder.

Reflexologists have identified ten energy channels beginning in the toes and extending to the fingers and top of the head. Each channel relates to a particular bodily zone, and to the organs in that zone. For example, the big toe relates to the head, i.e. the brain, ears, sinus area, neck, pituitary glands and eyes. By applying pressure to the appropriate terminal in the form of a small, specialized massage, a practitioner can determine which energy pathways are blocked.

Experts in this type of manipulative therapy claim that all the organs of the body are reflected in the feet. They also believe that reflexology aids the removal of waste products and blockages within the energy channels, improving circulation and gland function. Reflexology is certainly relaxing – for the mind and body. Indeed, as well as reducing stress, it can improve depression. Reportedly, like Indian head massage, it can increase the circulation of fluids in the head, and as such can be of benefit to individuals with sensorineural hearing loss.

Many therapists prefer to take down a full case history before commencing treatment. Each session will take up to forty-five minutes (the preliminary session may take longer), and you will be treated sitting in a chair or lying down.

Herbal remedies

Traditional Chinese herbal remedies have been used, to great effect, since antiquity – and are still the most widely used medicines in the world. In fact, 30 per cent of modern conventional medicines are made from plant-derived substances.

Although they are natural and there is a lower incidence of serious reactions than to conventional medications, herbal medicines should still be used with caution. Most are gentle and unlikely to cause serious side effects – but because, like conventional medication, they contain physiologically active agents, side effects can occur. The most common reactions are throat irritations, gastrointestinal upsets and headaches. You should always inform your GP, audiologist or ENT specialist of what you are taking. Indeed, many medical professionals believe herbal medicine should not be taken without the advice of a trained herbalist. Your chosen herbalist will check your pulse rate and the colour of your tongue for clues as to which bodily organs are energy-depleted. They will then write a prescription for very precise dosages according to your needs. Tablets made from compressed herbal extracts are often supplied, but sometimes patients are given a bag of carefully weighed and ground dried roots, flowers, bark and so on, together with instructions.

The herbs described below are considered useful for treating hearing impairment and tinnitus. Please note, however, that because there is often no dosage information for remedies purchased from a health shop or supermarket, it's difficult to know how much is too much. If you are taking large doses of prescription medication for severe symptoms, you may prefer to use herbal remedies for the more routine ailments you encounter.

Echinacea

One of the most researched herbs, echinacea has broad antibiotic properties, much like penicillin. It acts as an immune system stimulant, aids the destruction of germs and is capable of strengthening cell defences. As an antiviral agent, echinacea may be used by people who suffer from frequent ear infections, at first indications of such an infection. This may prevent a further decline in hearing. Adverse reactions are possible, so use carefully at first to monitor the effects.

Alcohol-free echinacea tinctures are now available from most health food shops. Alternatively, dry echinacea root – also available in health food shops – can be infused to make tea.

Goldenseal

Although there have been few studies into the effectiveness of goldenseal, it seems to work well when taken by mouth to treat the common cold, a stuffy nose and ear infections. Place half a dropperful of alcohol-free goldenseal extract in your mouth and swish it around for a few minutes before swallowing. Do this every three hours for three days. Alternating echinacea with goldenseal is said to work wonders.

Please note, however, that goldenseal should not be taken on a daily basis for more than one week at a time, and not used during pregnancy. This herb contains chemicals that may cause the muscles of the uterus to tighten, which may trigger a miscarriage. In addition, the alkaloids in goldenseal can pass into breast milk causing a potentially severe condition known as *kernicterus*, in which bile pigment builds up in the child's brain. Nursing mothers, therefore, should not use it. Moreover, if you have a history of cardiovascular disease, diabetes, or glaucoma, only use this herb under the supervision of your GP.

Garlic

This herb is useful for fighting viral, bacterial and parasitic infection, so can be of great benefit if you suffer from repeated infections of the ear or sinus tract. Garlic pearls are available from most health food shops. However, you may prefer to use natural garlic in your cooking.

To alleviate pain of the outer ear or ear canal, place a few drops of warm garlic oil or olive oil in the ear, then a drop or two of lobelia or mullein oil. You can plug the ear loosely with a cotton wool ball. If you are suffering from an infection of the middle or inner ear, you must seek medical attention. Your GP may still allow you to self-treat as a supplement to prescribed medication.

Onion poultice

Onion poultices can reduce the pain and shorten the life of outer ear and ear canal infections. To make an onion poultice, place a finely chopped onion between two pieces of cloth, rather than placing it in direct contact with the skin. Now hold to the ear for an hour or so. Alternatively, you could place the poultice between your ear and an old pillow when you go to bed at night – the smell of onions is likely to permeate the pillow.

For middle and inner ear infections, medical help must be sought. Your GP may give you permission to use an onion poultice as an adjunct to prescribed medication.

Ginkgo biloba

In the last 30 years, more that 300 studies have given clinical evidence that ginkgo biloba can be of benefit to many health problems throughout the human body. This herbal antioxidant is gaining recognition as a brain tonic that enhances memory because of its positive effects on the vascular system, especially in the cerebellum. It is also used as a treatment of vertigo and a variety of neurological and circulatory problems. The effects of ageing, including mental fatigue, lack of energy and hearing impairment can be counteracted by taking ginkgo biloba. Indeed, improvements in age-related hearing loss have been noted in clinical trials.

When a number of clinical trials investigating the effects of ginkgo biloba on tinnitus management were evaluated, it was found that there was a statistically significantly improvement – particularly when the tinnitus was due to reduced blood flow around the brain or disorders of the labyrinths of the ear. Further investigations showed that short-standing disorders, including hearing impairment and tinnitus, stand a better chance of improvement when treatment is begun early.

However, there have been other randomized controlled trials that indicate that ginkgo biloba is in fact ineffective in the treatment of tinnitus. For instance, in 1997, researchers conducted a double-blind placebo controlled trial of 99 subjects. The experimental group received 120 mg of ginkgo for a total of 12 weeks. A very small and non-statistically significant improvement in tinnitus was seen in the experimental group. This study was further expanded in 2001, stretching to a thousand subjects. The experimental group similarly received 150 mg of ginkgo biloba for a total of twelve weeks. Again, there was no statistically significant difference between the two groups. Experts now believe that insufficient quantities of ginkgo biloba were used, which could account for the negative result.

Ginkgo biloba can be purchased in capsule form from health food shops, some pharmacies and the larger supermarkets, and the label dosage instructions should be followed. Don't take ginkgo biloba if you are on warfarin, heparin or aspirin. Such drugs can react adversely to this supplement.

Rhodiola Rosea

This powerful Russian nutrient also belongs to the family of *adaptogenic* herbs – meaning a herb that can encourage a stressed body to adapt. Most health food shops now stock this stress-busting adaptogen, as do specialist supplement manufacturers (see Useful Addresses). Follow the label dosage instructions very carefully.

Ashwagandha

Also an adaptogenic herb, ashwagandha – sometimes called Indian ginseng – is an important tonic, containing a broad range of important healing powers rare in the plant kingdom. It has also been shown in research to help ease insomnia and stress.

In a study of 101 subjects, the indications of ageing – such as greying hair, low calcium levels and a deterioration in hearing – were found to be significantly improved in those taking ashwaganda (Kuppurajan, 1980).

Ashwagandha can be found in most health food shops and is available from specialist supplement manufacturers. Again, follow the label dosage instructions very carefully.

St John's Wort

St John's Wort is probably the most successful natural anti-depressant. Studies have shown that it works by increasing the action of the chemical serotonin and by inhibiting depression-promoting enzymes. Similar effects are created by the Prozac and Nardil families of chemical anti-depressants – both of which carry a high risk of side effects. St John's Wort, however, has the happy advantage of being virtually side effect free. In some cases it can produce a stomach upset, but this should stop within a few days.

One study has indicated that St John's Wort encourages sleep, and another that it benefits the immune system. In Germany, this herb outsells Prozac by three to one, and is said to be just as effective for treating mild depression. Because of its anti-inflammatory and antiviral properties, it can also be useful for treating ear infections.

(Note that because your skin may be more sensitive to the sun's rays when you are taking this herb, don't forget to use a good sun-block.)

Hopi ear candling (not recommended)

The practice of Hopi ear candling – also called thermal auricular therapy – involves lighting a hollow candle and placing it into the external auditory canal – the 'inner' part of the ear that's visible from the outside. It's said that such a lighted candle can create a vacuum that draws earwax (*cerumen*) and other impurities from the external auditory canal and deposits them in the candle as it burns. Some of the claimed benefits of ear candles include relieving sinus pressure and pain, curing ear infections and stopping tinnitus and vertigo.

However, it's important to note that when scientific research was carried out, it was established that ear candling could cause far more harm than good. The pressure generated by candling has actually been measured, and it was found to be absolutely nil, and analysis of the dark substance deposited in the candle revealed that it was candle wax, not earwax – which is not surprising.

Auditory specialists have reported treating the following problems, which have all arisen as a result of Hopi ear candle use:

- burns arising in the auricular and external auditory canal;
- blockage of the ear canal with candle wax;
- infection of the outer ear (*otitis externa*);
- perforation of the tympanic membrane.

Relaxation and meditation

Hearing impairment is likely to give rise to long-term frustration and anxiety, which leads to chronic stress – and chronic stress is the state of being constantly 'on alert'. The physiological changes associated with this state – a fast heart-rate, shallow breathing and muscular tension – often persist over a long period, making relaxation very difficult.

Chronic stress can lead to nerviness, hypertension, irritability and depression.

Deep breathing

In normal breathing, we take oxygen from the atmosphere down into our lungs. The diaphragm contracts and air is pulled into the chest cavity. When we breathe out, we expel carbon dioxide and other waste gases back into the atmosphere. But when we are stressed or upset, we tend to use the rib muscles to expand the chest. We breathe more quickly, sucking in shallowly. This is excellent in a crisis as it allows us to obtain the optimum amount of oxygen in the shortest possible time, providing our bodies with the extra power needed to handle the emergency. Some people do tend to get stuck in chest-breathing mode, however. Long-term shallow breathing is not only detrimental to physical and emotional health, it can also lead to hyperventilation, panic attacks, chest pains, dizziness and gastro-intestinal problems.

To test your breathing, ask yourself:

- How fast are you breathing as you are reading this?
- Are you pausing between breaths?
- Are you breathing with your chest or with your diaphragm?

A breathing exercise

The following deep breathing exercise should, ideally, be performed daily:

1 Make yourself comfortable in a warm room where you know you will be alone for at least half an hour.
2 Close your eyes and try to relax.
3 Gradually slow down your breathing, inhaling and exhaling as evenly as possible.
4 Place one hand on your chest and the other on your abdomen, just below your rib-cage.
5 As you inhale, allow your abdomen to swell upwards. (Your chest should barely move).
6 As you exhale, let your abdomen flatten.

Give yourself a few minutes to get into a smooth, easy rhythm. As worries and distractions arise, don't hang on to them. Wait calmly for them to float out of your mind – then focus once more on your breathing.

When you feel ready to end the exercise, open your eyes. Allow yourself time to become alert before getting up. With practice, you will begin breathing with your diaphragm quite naturally – and in times of stress, you should be able to correct your breathing without too much effort.

A relaxation exercise

Relaxation is one of the forgotten skills in today's hectic world, but it can help to counter the effects of the stress arising from hearing loss and tinnitus. It's advisable, therefore, that you learn at least one relaxation technique.

The following exercise is perhaps the easiest:

1 Make yourself comfortable in a place where you will not be disturbed. (Listening to restful music may help you relax.)
2 Begin to slow down your breathing, inhaling through your nose to a count of two.
3 Ensuring that the abdomen pushes outwards (as explained above), exhale to a count of four, five or six ...

After a couple of minutes, concentrate on each part of your body in turn, starting with your right arm. Consciously relax each set of muscles, allowing the tension to flow right out ... Let your arm feel heavier and heavier as every last remnant of tension seeps away ... Follow this procedure with the muscles of your left arm, then the muscles of your face, your neck, your stomach, your hips, and finally your legs.

Visualization

At this point, visualization can be introduced into the exercise. As you continue to breathe slowly and evenly, imagine yourself surrounded, perhaps, by lush, peaceful countryside, beside a gently trickling stream – or maybe on a deserted tropical beach, beneath swaying palm fronds, listening to the sounds of the ocean, thousands of miles from your worries and cares. Let the warm sun, the gentle breeze, the peacefulness of it all wash over you ...

The tranquillity you feel at this stage can be enhanced by repeating the exercise frequently – once or twice a day is best. With time, you should be able to switch into a calm state of mind whenever you feel stressed.

Meditation

Arguably the oldest natural therapy, meditation is the simplest and most effective form of self-help. Dr Herbert Benson of Harvard Medical School has been able to show that meditation tends to normalize blood pressure, the pulse rate and level of stress hormones in the blood. He has also proved that it produces changes in brain wave patterns, showing less excitability, and that it strengthens the immune system and endocrine system (hormones).

The unusual thing about meditation is that it involves 'letting go', allowing the mind to roam freely. Most of us are used to trying to control our thoughts – in our work, for example – so letting go is not as easy as it sounds.

It may help to know that people who regularly meditate say they have more energy, require less sleep, are less anxious, and feel far 'more alive' than before they did so. Ideally, the technique should be taught by a teacher – but as meditation is essentially performed alone, it can be learned alone with equal success.

Meditation may, to some people, sound a bit offbeat. But isn't it worth a try – especially when you can do it for free! Kick off those shoes and make yourself comfortable, somewhere you can be alone for a while. Now follow these simple instructions:

1 Close your eyes, relax, and practise the deep breathing exercise described above.

2 Concentrate on your breathing. Try to free your mind of conscious control.

3 Letting it roam unchecked, try to allow the deeper, more serene part of you to take over.

4 If you wish to go further into meditation, concentrate on mentally repeating a mantra – a certain word or phrase. It should be something positive, such as 'relax', 'I feel calm' or even 'I am special'.

5 When you are ready to finish, open your eyes and allow yourself time to adjust to the outside world before getting to your feet.

The aim of mentally repeating a mantra is to plant positive thoughts in your subconscious mind. It is a form of self-hypnosis, only you alone control the messages placed there.

Useful addresses

United Kingdom

British Tinnitus Association (BTA)
Ground Floor
Unit 5, Acorn Business Park
Woodseats Close
Sheffield S8 0TB
Freephone: 0800 018 0527
Fax: 0114 258 2279
Website: www.tinnitus.org.uk
Email: info@tinnitus.org.uk

This membership-based association is a registered charity supported by a team of eminent professional tinnitus advisers. It provides a quarterly magazine, *Quiet*, telephone support and details of 50 local tinnitus support groups.

Deafness Research UK (The Hearing Research Trust)
330–332 Gray's Inn Road
London WC1X 8EE
Tel.: 020 7833 1733
Freephone: 0808 808 2222
Text: 020 7915 1412
Fax: 020 7278 0404
Website: www.deafnessresearch.org.uk
Email: contact@deafnessresearch.org.uk

This organization is a medical charity for deaf and hard of hearing people. Its members aim to secure radical improvements in the prevention, diagnosis and treatment of all forms of hearing impairment, with the ultimate intention of finding cures for these distressing and neglected disabilities.

Hearing Aid Council (HAC)
70 St Mary Axe
London EC3A 8BD

Tel.: 020 3102 4030
Fax: 020 3102 4476
Website: www.thehearingaidcouncil.org.uk
Email: hac@thehearingaidcouncil.org.uk

Royal National Institute for Deaf People (RNID)
Head Office
19–23 Featherstone Street
London EC1Y 8SL
Tel.: 020 7296 8000
Textphone: 020 7296 8001
Fax: 020 7296 8199
Website: www.rnid.org.uk
Email: informationline@rnid.org.uk

The RNID is the largest charity working to change the world for the
UK's nine million deaf and hard of hearing people. Its website is
very thorough, containing advice and information for people with
hearing loss and tinnitus, and details of regional offices. There is
also detailed information about analogue and digital hearing aids
and an explanation of the Disability Discrimination Act and what it
means for you. You can also take a free hearing test by ringing 0845
600 5555. Details of the RNID online shop are given below.

Royal National Institute for Deaf People (RNID)
Products Team
1 Haddonbrook Centre
Orton Southgate
Peterborough PE2 6YX
Tel.: 0800 789 8855
Textphone: 01733 238 020
Fax: 0870 789 8822
Website: www.rnid.org.uk/shop
Email: solutions@rnid.org.uk

The RNID products team is responsible for the sale of products and
equipment for people with deafness, hearing loss and tinnitus via
the online shop and *Solutions* catalogue.

Australia

Australian Hearing
126 Greville Street
Chatswood
New South Wales 2067
Tel.: (02) 9412 6800
Textphone: (02) 9412 6802
Fax: (02) 9413 3855
Website: www.hearing.com.au

This web-based organization is dedicated to helping people to manage their hearing loss. It provides information, advice, links to similar organizations in other Australian states, and a full range of hearing services.

Tinnitus Association of Victoria
c/o Better Hearing Advisory Centre
5 High Street
Prahran
Victoria 3181
Tel.: (03) 9510 1577
Fax: (03) 9510 6076
Website: www.tinnitusvic.asn.au

This is a non-profit volunteer organization that provides a support network for tinnitus sufferers and their families.

Canada

The Canadian Hearing Society
271 Spadina Road
Toronto
Ontario M5R 2V3
Tel.: (416) 928 2500
Textphone: (416) 964 0023
Fax: (416) 928 2525
Website: www.chs.ca

This membership-based society, with regional branches all over the country, provides a variety of services, in English and French, that enhance the independence of deaf or hard of hearing people.

USA

Alexander Graham Bell Association for the Deaf and Hard of Hearing
3417 Volta Place, NW
Washington DC 20007
Tel.: (202) 337 5220
Website: www.agbell.org

This is a membership-based organization that aims to be a lifelong resource, support network and advocate for listening, learning, talking and living independently with hearing loss. The organization promotes the use of the spoken language and hearing technology through publications, advocacy, training, scholarships and financial aid.

American Tinnitus Association
PO Box 5
Portland
Oregon 97207 0005
Tel.: (800) 634 8978 (Toll Free within the United States)
Textphone: (503) 248 9985
Fax: (503) 248 0024
Website: www.ata.org
Email: tinnitus@ata.org

This is a non-profit-making organization with private funding that describes itself as a national champion of tinnitus research. Its four programme areas include education, advocacy, research and support. The association also facilitates self-help groups around the USA.

Hearing Loss Association of America
7910 Woodmont Avenue, Suite 1200
Bethesda
Maryland 20814
Tel.: (301) 657 2248

Fax: (301) 913 9413
Website: www.hearingloss.org
Email: information@hearingloss.org

This establishment describes itself as America's voice for people with hearing loss. It offers information and advice to sufferers and carers.

League for the Hard of Hearing

50 Broadway, 6th Floor
New York 10004
Tel.: (917) 305 7700 (voice)
       (917) 305 7999 (telephone typewriter – TTY)
Fax: (917) 305 7888
Website: www.lhh.org
Email: info@lhh.org

For information and advice on hearing issues, and also for free hearing screening.

National Association for the Deaf (NAD)

8630 Fenton Street, Suite 820
Silver Spring
Maryland 20910 3876
Tel.: (301) 587 1788 (Voice)
       (301) 587 1789 (TTY)
Fax: (301) 587 1791
Website: www.nad.org
Email: NADinfo@nad.org

The NAD works hard to make America a better place for all deaf and hard of hearing people. It does this by meeting an array of needs, emergencies and issues through position statements, legal statements, advisory letters to federal agencies and information materials. If you have access to the internet and would like to become a member, you can go to www.nad.org/join.

Other useful organizations

International Stress Management Association UK
PO Box 26
South Petherton
TA13 5WY
Tel.: 07000 780430
Website: www.isma.org.uk

This is a registered charity that exists to promote sound knowledge and best practice in the prevention and reduction of human stress.

DigiFocus II
Oticon Canada
10-7475 Kimbel Street
Mississauga
Ontario L5S 1E7
Canada
Tel.: (800) 263 8700
Fax: (905) 677 7760
Website: digifocus.oticon.ca
Email: general@oticon.ca

Oticon Canada sells the 100-per-cent digital and fully automatic hearing aid known as the DigiFocus II. This aid provides revolutionary sound quality, improving your ability to understand speech in the widest possible variety of listening situations. Its most important benefit is that it makes speech come through more clearly, so that you can feel more confident in social situations. Your audiology department may be able to order this aid for you.

Oticon Ltd (England)
Sales Office
Suite 1.7
Regent House
1–3 Queensway
Redhill
Surrey RH1 1QT
Tel.: 01737 734 860
Fax: 01737 734 861

Website: www.digifocus.oticon.co.uk
Email: info@oticon.co.uk

Oticon Ltd (Scotland)
Manufacturing Unit
PO Box 20
Hamilton
Lanarkshire ML3 7QE
Tel.: 01698 283363
Fax: 01698 284308
Website: www.digifocus.oticon.co.uk
Email: info@oticon.co.uk

Tinnitronics GmbH
Fuhrmannsgasse 8
A–1080 Wien
Austria
Tel.: +43 (0) 1 3679613
Fax: +43 (0) 1 3679615
Website: www.ti-ex.com
Email: office@ti-ex.com

This company provides information, in English and German, about tinnitus and the Ti-ex hearing device, which is comfortable to wear and allows magnetic fields to flow towards the damaged areas of the ear, giving relief to tinnitus sufferers. The device has been supplied to more than 50 countries.

References and further reading

References

Abel, S. M., et al., 'A study of acupuncture in adult sensorineural hearing loss'. *Journal of Otolaryngology*, 1976, 6 (2), pp. 166–72.

Cruickshanks, K. J., et al., 'Cigarette Smoking and Hearing Loss: The Epidemiology of Hearing Loss Study'. *Journal of American Medicine Association*, 1998, 279 (21), pp. 1715–19.

Kuppurajan, K., et al., 'Effect of Ashwagandha on the process of ageing in human volunteers'. *Journal of Research in Ayurveda and Siddha*, 1980, 1 (2), pp. 247–58.

Further reading

Burkey, John M., *Baby Boomers and Hearing Loss: A Guide to Prevention and Care*. Rutgers University Press, Chapel Hill, N.C., 2006.

Harvey, Michael A., *Odyssey of Hearing Loss: Tales of Triumph*. Dawn Sign Press, San Diego, Calif., 2003.

Hogan, Kevin, *Tinnitus, Turning the Volume Down: Proven Strategies for Quieting the Noise in Your Head*. Network 3000 Publishing, Eagan, Minn., 2003.

Jeffers, Janet, *Speechreading (Lipreading)*. Charles C. Thomas Publications, Springfield, Ill., 1980.

Lewycka, Marina, *Caring for Someone with a Hearing Loss* (Carers' Handbook Series). Age Concern, London, 2003.

Simmons, Michael, *Hearing Loss: From Stigma to Strategy*. Peter Owen, Chester Springs, Penn., 2005.

Yanick, Paul, *Natural Relief from Tinnitus: A Good Health Guide* (pamphlet). Keats Publications Inc., New Canaan, Conn., 2006.

Index